HORMONES,
HOT FLASHES and
MOOD SWINGS

ALSO BY THE AUTHOR

Your Pregnancy Month by Month

Primelife Pregnancy

HORMONES, HOT FLASHES and MOOD SWINGS

Living Through the Ups and Downs of Menopause

CLARK GILLESPIE, M.D.

PERENNIAL LIBRARY

HARPER & ROW, PUBLISHERS, NEW YORK
GRAND RAPIDS, PHILADELPHIA, ST. LOUIS, SAN FRANCISCO
LONDON, SINGAPORE, SYDNEY, TOKYO

Grateful acknowledgment is made to John Johnson Ltd. for permission to reprint "Warning," © Jenny Joseph, from *Rose in the Afternoon,* Dent, 1974.

FIRST EDITION

Designed by Barbara DuPree Knowles

Library of Congress Cataloging-in-Publication Data
Gillespie, Clark.
    Hormones, hot flashes, and mood swings : living through the ups and downs of menopause / Clark Gillespie.—1st ed.
        p.   cm.
    Includes index.
    ISBN 0-06-055162-3 : $.—ISBN 0-06-096355-7 (pbk.) : $
    1. Menopause—Popular works.   I. Title.
RG186.G54   1989   88-45934
618.1'75—dc20   CIP

---

89 90 91 92 93 CC/FG 10 9 8 7 6 5 4 3 2
    91 92 93 CC/FG 10 9 8 7 6   (pbk.)

FOR MY BELOVED WIFE, *Susan*

When I am an old woman I shall wear purple
With a red hat which doesn't go, and doesn't suit me.
And I shall spend my pension on brandy and summer gloves
And satin sandals and say we've no money for butter.
I shall sit down on the pavement when I'm tired
And gobble up samples in shops and press alarm bells
And run my stick along the public railings
And make up for the sobriety of my youth.
I shall go out in my slippers in the rain
And pick the flowers in other people's gardens
And learn to spit . . .
But maybe I ought to practise a little now?
So people who know me are not too shocked and surprised
When suddenly I am old, and start to wear purple.

—JENNY JOSEPH

Contents

Introduction

Four facts relating to women and aging have now become abundantly and unequivocally clear. First, life expectancy for women has increased dramatically in the United States during this century. Second, women are not only living longer, but are living healthier lives. This is due in part to improved lifestyles and in part to quality lifetime medical care, which has mitigated many of the potentially lethal and crippling disorders that at one time commonly afflicted women. Third, a fresh, reasonably healthy four million recruits are added each year to the more than forty million women presently living in the menopausal continuum. And one woman in seven will be over sixty-five by the turn of the century. All menopausal women will, of course, pass on. But that moment is being pushed farther away all the time, and as a result the menopausal and postmenopausal society continues to grow. Finally, and most important, menopause and the years that follow have been clearly established as an endocrine deficiency state—a disorder worthy of, and indeed, almost always requiring, comprehensive treatment.

Based on the preceding facts, this handbook has been written for, and is addressed to, all those women struggling through the menopause years. It is to serve as a companion and guide while you experience this tremendous journey— which, like all explorations, has its peaks and valleys, dangers and delights, dead ends and vistas, and which, without compass points, can lead to arid sand and stone rather than milk, honey and wine. Very clearly, these years can be savored or suffered, depending upon the route with which you are provided and whether or not you choose to follow it. The menopausal journey is a continuous one—always slightly uphill or downhill, but with some neat plateaus. In these pages I try to provide a gentle and compassionate compass for your journey.

HORMONES,
HOT FLASHES and
MOOD SWINGS

CHAPTER ONE

The Fruitful Years

The human menstrual life can be compared, with safety, to the life of a rose. Both lie dormant as the host grows, begin to bud in the exuberance of youth, flower in the fullness of adulthood, bear fruit for generation, and then draw back to support newer buds along the stem. And although a rose is supposedly sweeter in the bud than in full bloom, nothing is more exquisite than the fragrance of an open rose—particularly an open autumn rose—and, not to prolong the floral allegory further, long after the bloom is off the rose, the attar of its petals lives on to perfume the days of winter.

The Beginning

Stimulated by our great master gland, the pituitary, menstrual life sputters and starts as little girls begin to become young women. The rose buds as follows:

In about the ninth year of a girl's life the pituitary gland begins to awaken both ovaries by emitting two powerful hormones—*FSH (follicle stimulating hormone)* and *LH (luteinizing hormone).*

FSH stimulates one or more of the thousands of immature eggs (follicles) in the ovaries to begin a maturation cycle. Although it may be several years before *ovulation,* the process in which one maturing egg ruptures from the ovarian capsule and follows its course, FSH induces the maturing eggs to begin to secrete *estrogen,* the primary female hormone. Mainly under the influence of estrogen, genital maturation begins. This maturation includes growth and development of the secondary sexual apparatus, such as the breasts and thighs, and the primary apparatus, which includes the vagina along with the uterus and its lining, the *endometrium.* The endometrium begins to undergo cyclical changes and menstruation begins (menarche) even before regular ovulation takes place.

LH sooner or later forces *ovulation* (see glossary) to take place, and a physiological cyst called the *corpus luteum* forms where ovulation has occurred. This cyst secretes the hormone *progesterone,* which, among many other things, prepares the endometrium (during a 14-day term) for a fertilized egg. If none arrives, the corpus luteum shrinks and stops making progesterone, the endometrium withers, and menstruation (menses) occurs. Ovulation begins 14 days after the onset of the last menstrual period. And so it goes, more or less regularly, every 28 days, unless pregnancy intervenes. If it does, the corpus luteum lives on, continuing to make the progesterone which, in turn, continues to nurture the endometrium, and so menstruation does not take place. Thus, the very first sign of pregnancy. No period.

Unless interrupted by pregnancy or some other phenomenon, this regular cycle continues until the menopause. There are many problems associated with menstruation. Not all of them are dealt with in this handbook. Some, however, are related to the menopause and thus become our problems, and they will have their moment with us.

The Menopause

The menopause is likely to come upon you as you approach your middle forties—but before we get into it here, some terms need to be defined.

Menopause. This is what our book is all about—but few people can agree upon what the menopause actually is. *MPX* is a medical abbreviation for "menopause," and we will use it often. The word was coined by a Frenchman from Greek words meaning, roughly, end of monthlies. But in modern usage it has become synonymous with all the events that take place as the ovaries cease to function. Thus, the interruption, irregularity or cessation of periods and the attendant emotional and physical changes—some of which (bone calcium loss, for instance) continue to be an influence for the remainder of life—are all considered to be "menopausal" and part of the total "menopausal complex." And that is the way menopause will be considered in our handbook—the beginning of the great adventure.

Climacteric. This term includes all the emotional and physical changes that take place as ovarian function diminishes—but it does not necessarily include the physical cessation of menstrual periods. Thus, the climacteric embraces such symptoms as flushes, night sweats, insomnia, emotional instability, depression, fatigue, forgetfulness, palpitations, and so forth. The climacteric ceases—by definition—in a few years. The *change of life* might be considered synonymous with the climacteric.

Perimenopause. The years that immediately precede the menopause are called the perimenopause (PeriMPX). At this time the *premenstrual syndrome* (described below) is likely to be exaggerated. Moreover, even while menstruation remains reasonably regular, menopausal symptoms often are felt. Thus, flushes, night sweats, palpitations, emotional instability, forgetfulness and more are not uncommon at this time and will accelerate as the menopause moves along.

Postmenopause. From the time that ovarian function ceases more or less completely (but never quite completely, unless the ovaries are diseased or removed surgically), women enter their postmenopausal life. Without hormone replacement, the postmenopausal (PMPX) years usually consist of a continuous gradual decline in physical and emotional function.

Premature (early) menopause. When a woman's ovarian function declines early in life—anytime before she reaches the age of forty—a premature menopause exists. It may be temporary (because of illness, strenuous physical activity, stress, etc.) or permanent (resulting from removal of the ovaries, a familial or autoimmune disorder, or destructive ovarian disease). Whether temporary or permanent, typical menopausal symptoms occur.

Premenstrual syndrome (PMS). Existing since the beginning of time but only recently legitimized, this condition is characterized by certain emotional and physical changes that precede each menstruation by a few days to a week. Commonly, there is retention of fluid (swelling, edema), breast tenderness, headaches, irritability, emotional instability, depression, fatigue, lassitude, insomnia and considerably more. Many women aptly refer to this distressing cycle of events as a Jekyll-Hyde existence. The PMS tends to deepen and to last longer as the perimenopause deepens and the menopause approaches.

As a general pattern, ovarian function begins to decline somewhere between forty-five and fifty. The ovaries run out of eggs that are capable of maturation and hormone production and, as a result, the pituitary gland, recognizing the ovarian decline, emits exceedingly high levels of FSH to try to get the ovaries' attention. It doesn't work—at least not for long—and ovarian function, ovulation, and hormone production all diminish. The loss of ovarian progesterone and then estrogen leaves the endometrium without adequate nourishment, and so menstruation becomes erratic and eventually ceases.

The loss of *progesterone* causes several changes, including a few problems:

• There *may* be a temporary decrease in premenstrual symptoms.

• Irregular and abnormal periods are much more likely to occur.

• If estrogen secretion continues (even in small amounts) in the absence of progesterone, cancer of the endometrium, and perhaps of the breasts, is more likely to take place down the line. As we shall see, small amounts of estrogen may continue to be present and function in the body during the post-menopausal years by a variety of mechanisms. Without progesterone to complement it in certain tissues, unopposed estrogen can become a serious malignant irritant.

When *significant* regular *estrogen* production ceases, for whatever reason, very important bodily changes are set in motion:

• The endometrium ceases to grow; it becomes *atrophic* (begins to waste away).

• The uterus begins to shrivel, ending up one-half its active size.

• The vagina also undergoes aging changes. First, its lining skin becomes thin and dry, and loses elasticity and resiliency. The skin appears to be shiny or waxy. Infections are more likely to take place and sexual pain is common. Lubrication is absent.

• Like the vagina, the external genitalia (vulva) become thin, waxy and more subject to irritation and diseases. Lubricating glands stop secreting and the skin is therefore more likely to crack when stretched or irritated. In time, the clitoris may become encased in thinning skin, becoming less accessible and responding more slowly—or not at all—to sexual stimulation.

• During the decline in estrogen production, breast tenderness may temporarily increase. Eventually the breasts wither as glandular tissue becomes inactive.

• Generally, all body skin becomes thin and dry. Thus, wrinkling increases and superficial blood vessels appear more prominently. Often the skin darkens, and brown aging spots appear along with dark hair.

• In the absence of estrogen, bone loss accelerates; susceptible women can lose as much as 2 percent of their bone mass each year, producing in time *osteoporosis,* which now destroys more American women than cancer of the uterus and breast *combined.*

• Vasomotor responses in the brain affect the diameter of various blood vessels and are responsible for the "puffs of heat" that plague almost all menopausal women to varying degrees at some time or another. Without hormone replacement, flushes and sweats often persist for years.

• Much as with the premenstrual syndrome, depression, emotional instability, irritability, fatigue, lassitude and insomnia, and more regularly accompany the other symptoms of estrogen deprivation at the menopause.

• Significant sexual problems may be manifested at this stage and become progressively more severe as time goes on. Structurally, as we have seen, the vagina and vulva become thin and dry, prone to infection and likely to make intercourse painful. Moreover, sexual stimulation will not induce natural lubrication. The time it takes to reach orgasm is prolonged, and orgasm may eventually not be achieved at all. Finally, sexual drive is often reduced or evaporates.

• Without estrogen, arteriosclerosis hastens to clog important arteries. This degenerative change is accelerated in the presence of nicotine and excess blood lipids (fats). Thus, postmenopausal women begin to catch up to men in their rate of heart attacks and strokes.

All the above changes do take place as estrogen departs— some to greater degrees than others—depending upon a number of circumstances. These categories of estrogen deprivation will all be dealt with as this handbook proceeds on. One conclusion from all this, however, is inescapable: the menopause is a hormone deficiency disorder with massive medical and social implications. And it has been neglected too long.

◆§ *Pause and Reflect*

During her entire lifetime, a woman produces no more than one-fifth of an ounce of estrogen and progesterone—roughly 6 grams—or the amount of sugar you would put in your morning coffee. Talk about a concentrated sweetener!

All ovarian hormones are manufactured within the body from cholesterol—cholesterol that comes either from food intake or from synthesis within the liver. They are called *steroid* hormones (from the Greek *stereos,* meaning "solid") because, although they are members of the vast alcohol family, they will crystallize solid instead of evaporating. Structurally, they are all nearly identical, but, of course, physiologically they are marvelously unique from one other and in their effects upon the body. Incidentally, the male hormone testosterone is a member of the same steroid family, and almost identical to estrogen except that it has one molecule of water tacked on in an odd location. What a difference a little drink can make!

Lydia Bronte, Director of Carnegie Foundation's Aging Society project, was quoted recently as describing a new maturing age between fifty and seventy-five. Almost imperceptibly, this new stage of adult life has been developing and instead of being a time of decline and death, as it has been historically, it is now a new prime of life. Quoting her directly:

> *Age 65 is no longer a real watershed in physical and mental vigor. An underground and undocumented phenomenon is occurring. People in this age group are already pioneering new lifestyles and new patterns, with no previous models to guide them. They are a priceless resource for society.*

Where did the word "menopause" come from? I am going to tell you, and not only that—I am myself going to translate the two paragraphs of the dissertation given by Professor Gardanne (in Paris, 1812) in which he coined the word. This dissertation was where that word was first actually used.

Forgive my French.

> *The menstrual cessation has received many names: some calling it "the critical epoc," cessation of the monthly or regulars, others describing it as the disappearance of regulars, others as the disappearance of menses, the retreat of age, decline of age, winter of women, death of sex, the critical time, etc. Finally, one is lost in the profusion of names.*
>
> *The word "menopause" (ménépausie), I believe, expresses perfectly the ideas that one attaches to these diverse events; "menopause" is composed of two Greek words—"month" and "terminate."*

And there you have it.

CHAPTER TWO

Premature Menopause

T hings come and go, but not always on schedule. And so it is with normal rhythmic ovarian function. Unlike the cycles of the moon, the sun and the stars in their courses, regular ovarian function from the very onset is neither immutable, unshakable or totally predictable. Thus ovarian function may cease well before the expected forty-fifth year. And such a halt may signal temporary ovarian failure (TOF) or premature (and permanent) ovarian failure (POF).

Temporary Ovarian Failure

Temporary ovarian failure (TOF), like POF, begins with failure to ovulate (and thus no production of progesterone—remember?) and generally progresses until little or no ovarian hormone production exists at all. Thus, both estrogen and progesterone are absent. TOF implies that recovery can and does occur—generally with the elimination or control of the inciting cause or causes.

WHAT CAUSES TEMPORARY OVARIAN FAILURE?

Temporary ovarian failure may result from any of the following causes:

• *Stress.* Events or conditions that rob the body of internal homeostasis, or balance, very quickly affect the pituitary/ovary relationship and cause the ovaries to shut down. Stress is the commonest cause of TOF and any source of stress— good (traveling abroad) or bad (loss of a loved one)—can at least temporarily arrest ovarian function. Other common stresses include excessive physical activity (intense athletic training), anorexia, obesity, unemployment, and being in love, in arrears, or in debt. You may be aware of others.

• *Systemic disorders.* Particularly when they are out of control, systemic disorders can arrest ovarian function until recovery from the particular condition takes place. Thus, diabetes, hypertension (high blood pressure), anemia and other serious generalized disorders will produce TOF and amenorrhea (absence of menstruation). Chemotherapy and radiation for cancer have a similar depressive ovarian effect—and one that is not always temporary. Similarly, acute health problems such as serious surgery or infections often induce short-term TOF. If elevated, *prolactin,* a pituitary hormone, can also interrupt menstruation until the pituitary disorder responsible for its elevation is corrected. Ovulation, of course, ceases with this disorder. Certain disorders of the thyroid and adrenal glands can interrupt ovarian function until such disorders can be controlled.

• *Ovarian disease.* Certain ovarian tumors and infections will temporarily suppress normal ovarian function. As an example, an unusual masculinizing tumor of the ovaries usually first declares itself by bringing an end to menstruation. And there are others; they must all, of course, be successfully treated before ovarian function may resume.

• *Destructive habits.* The use of tobacco, alcohol and drugs and certain abnormal eating habits (bulemia, anorexia and malnutrition) all have a marked effect on ovarian activity and all can induce TOF and amenorrhea.

• *Birth control pills.* Oral contraceptives suppress ovulation and largely supplant ovarian function. When oral contraceptives are discontinued, the ovaries, shackled for so long, may hesitate before taking their first step toward regaining normal function. Once in a while, they need help.

THE DIAGNOSIS OF TEMPORARY OVARIAN FAILURE

How is TOF diagnosed? Although it may seem too obvious to mention, pregnancy must first be ruled out when a period—or a number of periods—are missed. A surprising number of unnecessary tests have been ordered due to this blind spot or diagnostic oversight. When pregnancy is confirmed by examination or laboratory testing, a new adventure begins somewhere else.

After pregnancy has been eliminated as a possible cause, a complete physical examination and regular laboratory studies are in order. Thus, any systemic disorder that might contribute to the ovarian failure can be identified. A *provocative* or *challenge progesterone test* is the most usual next step. A fixed dose of progesterone is administered either by mouth for seven days or by a single injection. Menstrual bleeding will follow within a few days or a few weeks *if* the ovaries have been secreting enough estrogen to prime the endometrium; the externally supplied progesterone completes the endometrial maturation and produces a period.

If a period *does* follow this challenge, we know that the endometrium is working and will respond to adequate hormone stimulation. It is not the cause of the menstrual cessation. We also know that the ovaries are failing to ovulate but are still producing estrogen. Failure is not complete.

If menstruation does not respond to the challenge, we then supply both estrogen and progesterone in a cyclic manner. A menstrual response following this degree of stimulation tells us that the endometrium is healthy, needing only hormone food for growth, and that ovarian failure is complete, since neither estrogen nor progesterone is being secreted.

Now we have established that ovarian failure exists. Is it temporary or permanent? Is it a disorder of the ovaries themselves (primary) or is it from an outside source (secondary)?

More testing is now necessary. Studies of pituitary, adrenal and thyroid gland function are all very relevant. The pituitary studies test FSH, LH and prolactin levels at the very least. Adrenal gland disorders that can interrupt menstruation are not uncommon and involve the abnormal production of both *cortisone* and certain other adrenal hormones with masculinizing characteristics; these hormone levels are tested as well. Tests are also taken to determine if increased or decreased thyroid functions have halted menses. Certain other thyroid (and adrenal, for that matter) tests may determine the presence of autoimmune disorders that also attack the ovaries. See Premature Ovarian Failure, beginning on page 16.

Further observations and studies are necessary to eliminate systemic disorders that may be working their will upon the ovaries. A genetic history and chromosomal studies may be indicated. Finally, biopsy of both ovaries under direct visualization (a surgical exploration) may have to be done.

By following the above outline (and there are many variations to this approach that are employed in different clinics), we can determine whether the ovarian failure is temporary or permanent and proceed with proper care. Let me hasten to say that many times a patient experiences menstrual cessation and the cause is so clear at that time that no intensive workup is indicated. Thus, an otherwise healthy 25-year-old woman in the throes of a difficult divorce, living on cigarettes and coffee, not menstruating and not pregnant, needs our help and not our workup. Menstruation will follow when she is through her troubled time. If it doesn't, then a study can be considered, but it is seldom necessary.

THE TREATMENT OF TEMPORARY OVARIAN FAILURE

The management of temporary ovarian failure is easy to outline. First, the doctor and patient must treat the cause, which may not be as simple as it sounds. Nevertheless, treatment should be directed toward the elimination of the offending cause. All the culprits described earlier will generally, sooner or later, yield to appropriate treatment and allow the ovaries to go about their normal business.

Second, *hormone replacement therapy (HRT)* may be necessary. The use of supplemental hormones during this period of temporary failure is generally indicated (unless the failure is extremely short-lived). HRT is important because symptoms of estrogen depletion—including flushes, insomnia and fatigue—are usually present and unpleasant; significant bone loss takes place in prolonged estrogen deprivation at any age; and the endometrium needs regular stimulation to keep it healthy.

HRT may consist of oral contraceptives or other estrogen-progesterone combinations (when oral contraceptives are contraindicated).

Premature Ovarian Failure

Premature ovarian failure (POF) is, by our definition, permanent and complete and represents or, indeed actually is, a premature menopause. It happens before the fortieth year and includes all the symptoms of estrogen deprivation: irregular, delayed menses followed by total cessation of periods; flushes; night sweats; insomnia; fatigue; emotional instability; vaginal dryness and more.

POF involves about 5 percent of all women under forty and is generally preceded by several years of irregular, delayed menses. For these women, the onset of puberty is generally normal but breast development may be depressed. Of the 5 percent of women involved, a third who enter this state of POF have never conceived and about one in ten has a family history of POF.

WHAT CAUSES PREMATURE OVARIAN FAILURE?

Genetic abnormalities are associated with 18 percent of all premature ovarian failure. Both abnormal sex chromosomes and abnormal regular chromosomes (autosomes) may induce a premature menopause. Women with POF caused by genetic abnormalities are usually short of stature, have a family history of POF, and have other congenital abnormalities that further assist in their clinical identification. Chromosome cultures may clearly identify this problem, but ovarian cell cultures may be necessary in a "mosaic" individual (one who has inherited and carries two distinct cell lines that may not be detected by routine genetic culturing). Thus, blood chromosome cultures may be normal but ovarian chromosome cultures may not.

Autoimmune disorders are responsible for at least 12 percent of all premature ovarian failure. Under these circumstances the body builds self-destructive antibodies to its own glandular system, causing a sort of polyglandular suicide. These antibodies, which are usually directed against the adrenal and thyroid glands, can also be detected, though only with considerable difficulty. Not every clinic can do it.

Defects in ovarian metabolism and function probably account for 12 percent of all POF. In this broad dysfunction, all of the proper eggs are present and in order but due to metabolic failure that is poorly understood, maturation does not take place and hormone secretion fails.

Ovarian damage from radiation, chemotherapy and infection, along with, of course, ovarian removal at surgery, eliminates all functions related to these glands. Ovarian damage accounts for 40 percent of all POF.

Acquired defects caused by viral disorders (mumps, for instance) particularly at the time of puberty, along with certain other systemic infections, are sometimes responsible for POF in later years. These defects account for 8 percent of POF.

All the remaining causes of POF—which account for about 10 percent of the total cases—are grouped in the unknown category. As time goes by, this category diminishes in size but will probably always exist.

THE DIAGNOSIS OF PREMATURE OVARIAN FAILURE

A great number of cases of premature ovarian failure can be identified through a medical history. A history of familial and inherited disorders, or of ovarian damage or removal, or of radiation or chemotherapy, or of many other causes can be elicited just by talking to the patient. Confirmatory evidence is easy to obtain.

Temporary ovarian failure must be eliminated by the procedures listed above.

Chromosome culturing and autoimmune testing can be done in appropriate clinical settings where such procedures are available. When they are not immediately available, blood specimens drawn in any office can generally be transferred to research laboratories capable of providing exact results in a reasonable period of time. Not always, though, at a reasonable price!

Ovarian biopsy may provide the definitive answer. Proper ovarian sampling taken directly and in adequate amounts will establish whether there is any finite pattern of ovarian life expectancy. The absence of follicles capable of maturation clearly indicates that ovarian function has permanently ceased.

THE TREATMENT OF PREMATURE OVARIAN FAILURE

Hormone replacement therapy is very important and should be instituted early. Early treatment can prevent osteoporosis, delay arteriosclerosis, prevent involution and atrophy of the sexual system and sexual drive, and allay early menopausal symptoms.

These needs all will be clearly explained as we move on. Along with HRT it is important to carry out all the other programs—diet, exercise, lifestyle and the like—that can be found in this book.

◄§ *Pause and Reflect*

By the twentieth week of gestation, a female fetus has 6 to 7 million immature eggs in her ovaries—the most she will ever have. At birth, about 1 million eggs remain, and at puberty, only 300,000 are left. Of these, only about 300 will mature and undergo ovulation during a normal lifetime. Thus 99.9 percent of all the eggs are lost along the way!

How the 300 eggs that will be released from the ovaries are awakened and committed to ovulation is not yet fully understood. The process is, however, relentless, and continues on whether ovulation is suppressed (by birth control pills, for instance) or not. Any process that diminishes the number of available immature follicles at puberty or hastens their death will hasten premature ovarian failure.

Recent studies of rodents have revealed some reproductive aging secrets. In one study, a group of young rats had their ovaries surgically removed. When the rats grew old, they had fresh young ovaries implanted and the rats began regular cyclic activity just as youngsters would! This piece of research might lead to techniques that allow human ovarian activity to be suspended—for whatever reason—and reactivated in later years. So can one have a baby at sixty? I doubt it. But important uses of such research may come in time. And our pool of knowledge grows—as does our indebtedness to fragile little animals.

CHAPTER THREE

The Premenstrual Syndrome and the Perimenopause

As surely as twilight precedes dusk, the premenstrual syndrome (PMS) precedes the perimenopause (PeriMPX). And, as surely as dusk is followed by nightfall, so the perimenopause is followed by the menopause (MPX). That is the way it all goes. Dusk, twilight, nightfall; premenstrual syndrome, perimenopause, menopause. It might have been better to compare this chain of menopausal events with daybreak, dawn and morning—but it's afternoon for us now.

At any rate, the ovarian hormone decline, which begins in the thirties, is simply a chain of unfolding events. It's helpful to review the terms we've used:

Premenstrual syndrome (PMS). In the first place, "syndrome" generally means that doctors are unsure of which symptoms and signs contribute to a disorder (and also that we doctors don't know much about it). But PMS generally precedes a menstrual period by seven to ten days and includes (but is not limited to) mood swings, depression, irritability, fatigue, lassitude, fluid retention, abdominal swelling, headaches and breast tenderness.

Perimenopause (PeriMPX). This is an arbitrary division of the continuing ovarian decline. It is useful to distinguish it from the PMS for treatment purposes. The PeriMPX begins a few years before the true menopause. It is characterized by longer and deeper PMS bites plus increasing menstrual irregularities, and often by the onset of flushes and insomnia, usually experienced just before the menses. In essence, so the PMS is the beginning of the beginning of the end and the PeriMPX is the beginning of the end of the menstrual cycle. There are many variations in the timing and extent of these symptoms in each individual, and as a result it is difficult to identify and separate these two conditions.

The Premenstrual Syndrome

No one knows the true cause of PMS and thus no one is privy to the correct treatment. Theories and therapies abound, but no one knows the cure. What are the theories? For what they're worth, here they are:

• *Psychological.* "It's all in the mind." This convenient and large pigeonhole has been stuffed by the medical profession from the beginning of time to dismiss any illness it could not, or would not, understand. Although some of us get every disease we read about—which is why the incidence of PMS is apparently increasing at the same rate as the consumption of newsprint—you can discount the "all in your mind" theory. Some can fantasize PMS but most feel it.

• *Hormonal.* As the thirties creep toward the forties, basic changes occur in the cyclic production of estrogen and progesterone in many women. These cyclic changes have been incriminated as the instigator of PMS.

But are these changes really at fault? Consider this: One night you drink scotch and soda and get drunk. Then the next night you drink bourbon and soda and again get drunk. If you know nothing about the ingredients—scotch, bourbon and soda—you swear that you will never drink soda again. It was the only thing you had *both* nights, and it made you drunk!

Silly? Maybe so, but a lot of PMS research has been conducted with no greater controls than those used in our whiskey experiment.

The fact that certain hormone changes may coincide with the blossoming of PMS does not therefore prove that one causes the other. There may be a relationship, but it is yet to be proven. And treatment of PMS with the hormones involved—estrogen and progesterone—has not been very successful.

• *Nutritional.* This once-popular theory held that PMS resulted when certain nutritional substances were in arrears. Amongst the most favored diet-lapses was (and still is) vitamin B_6. Unfortunately, replacement of this nutrient has not helped very many PMS sufferers. Also, excess salt, flour, white vinegar and caffeine have equally been accused, but to no avail. And so the search for causes goes on.

• *Abnormal pituitary/ovary interaction.* This is the most complicated theory of all—and therefore the least likely to be right. Involved in this theory are certain neuropeptides. These are messenger chemicals sent to cerebral headquarters from the ovaries that *demand* bitchiness and discomfort. Again, this is a theory and there is no sustaining proof.

• *Other.* Abnormalities of sugar metabolism, magnesium deficiency, prolactin disorders and prostaglandins (substances made in the uterus and certain other organs that can produce powerful uterine contractions) are some of the leading candidates for the "other" category. All of them fail to explain the whole PMS complex.

Regardless of which theory of origin is correct, certain things are very clear about PMS: It afflicts four out of five women to a *varying* degree; it is real—as real as the male mid-life crisis, prostatic hypertrophy (enlarged prostate) and impotence; and it increases in severity and duration as the perimenopause approaches, folding into it without a hitch.

SYMPTOMS OF THE PREMENSTRUAL SYNDROME

PMS has a triad of symptoms and not every woman experiences them all. The triad consists of: *altered emotions,* which include anxiety, depression, tension and irritability; *body changes,* which include weight gain, breast tenderness, bloating and edema, migraine, appetite increase and cravings, fatigue, constipation and palpitations; and *behavioral changes,* which include alterations in social contacts, work habits, coordination and sex drive.

THE DIAGNOSIS OF THE PREMENSTRUAL SYNDROME

Most often the diagnosis of PMS is made on the basis of history alone. There are few, if any, physical signs that confirm a diagnosis of PMS, although a complete physical examination is always recommended. Sometimes women are requested to keep a diary of their cyclic manifestations for several months. This not only helps to confirm the diagnosis but clearly indicates the duration of each monthly episode and the major symptoms. Present-day laboratory tests are of no diagnostic value at all, except to eliminate other systemic illnesses.

THE TREATMENT OF THE PREMENSTRUAL SYNDROME

Since there is no single known cause of PMS, there is no single treatment. Here, nevertheless, are some commonly employed treatment programs:

• *Altered lifestyle.* Many women are advised to alter their lifestyles during the PMS stress so as to avoid situations that will increase their tension and decrease their coping ability. In accordance with this recommendation, social, financial, familial and sexual confrontations should be pegged and post-dated. Such environmental manipulation involves the intense cooperation of most living-in loved ones. Husbands, mates, children and parents have to be provided with necessary intelligence and information so that they can assist in avoiding potential conflicts in your monthly cycle. This is a great time to procrastinate! Put off till tomorrow what will annoy you today.

• *Physical exercise.* Moderate physical activity on a regular basis and away from your home base is especially good if depression is a major component of PMS. It is good for you anyway. Low-impact aerobics, swimming, walking, cycling, tennis and so on help to reduce tension. This is one of the very best therapies.

• *Diet.* Cravings for sugar, salt, caffeine, and other food elements are not uncommon during PMS and none of these things help the situation. In fact, salt makes the swelling worse and caffeine makes the nerves worse. Sugar—well, you know about sugar.

To combat PMS, most nutritionists recommend frequent

small meals that include more complex carbohydrates. (See Diet, pages 75–84.)

• *Diuretics.* Edema or swelling of the extremities and the breasts, along with abdominal bloating, is one of the commonest companions of PMS. Often the intermittent use of appropriate diuretics (water pills) will help get rid of this unwanted water. The abuse of diuretics can be dangerous and counterproductive, so heed your doctor's advice.

• *Mood control.* Many psychotropic drugs have been used to help control the tension, depression, anxiety and insomnia that PMS breeds. These include tranquilizers, antidepressants, and anxiolytics. Recently, a program involving the controlled use of Xanax has been most successful.

• *Hormone replacement.* Since hormone imbalances of various sorts have been commonly incriminated as a major cause of PMS, it clearly follows that various hormone-juggling programs are recommended to manage PMS symptoms. These programs fall into two basic categories: estrogen leveling and progesterone supplements.

Some clinicians, who believe that wide swings in estrogen levels during a regular cycle is a fundamental contributor to PMS, advocate supplementing internal estrogen production in a variety of ways so that there are no estrogen peaks or pits.

A significant number of gynecologists believe that PMS is caused by a progesterone deficiency. Thus their therapy is directed toward increasing the levels of this hormone during the second half of the menstrual cycle. To this end they have devised a progesterone vaginal suppository as a mechanism to deliver pure progesterone during the last two weeks of each cycle. The suppository was developed because pure progesterone cannot be given orally and injections—on a long-term basis—are unwieldy. This work began in England and, although the suppositories are available in some parts of our country, they are not approved by the FDA for any legitimate medical purpose. That does not mean, however, that they are bad, useless or dangerous. It does mean that they are hard to come by.

In spite of the interest in hormonal therapy for the management of PMS, no controlled study has revealed a correlation between any hormone imbalance or deficiency and PMS. Further, no controlled clinical study has shown any consistent improvement of PMS on hormone therapy, or any improvement that is better than a placebo effect.

Because no one understands the cause of PMS, none of the suggested treatments have been overwhelmingly successful. In general, the results have been variable, unpredictable, and often unsatisfactory. There is little doubt, however, that dietary and lifestyle changes accompanied by an exercise program will help minimize the effects of this disabling syndrome.

The Perimenopause

You already know that the premenstrual syndrome flows inevitably into the perimenopause. Sooner or later, the one becomes the other. However, two things need to be reemphasized right now: First, not *all* women are significantly disturbed by the PMS and the PeriMPX. You should simply wait, let nature unfold, and see what comes along and has to be dealt with. Sometimes, like an IRS audit, nothing shows up.

Second, so ingrained is the double standard of aging that it can hardly fail to shake the confidence of the most mature, stable and secure woman. Women have to face not only what the menopause itself actually brings to them, but they must also face what cultures have added to it. As a result of all this interplay, significant psychological storms may now gather strength. It is important to keep these cultural factors in mind as you near the menopause.

You will remember that ovarian function is finite and that the ovaries are organs with a limited active life cycle. Although there are hundreds of thousands of immature follicles in each ovary, only a few hundred in a lifetime can ripen into mature eggs that are capable of being ovulated and fertilized. Moreover, if these eggs are not spent during the reproductive years, they cannot be saved and spent later.

As the ovaries age and the number of capable follicles diminishes, the pituitary gland signals the ovaries (with FSH, the follicle stimulating hormone) to get back to work. Alas, it is of little avail and gradually inferior follicles are stimulated. These marginal follicles produce estrogen as the eggs struggle to mature, but the eggs are incapable of undergoing ovulation. Thus, no progesterone is released and cyclic menstrual bleeding will, as a result, inevitably change. Moreover, the amount of estrogen produced in each cycle will gradually decline, so symptoms of estrogen deficiency will begin to appear. Sometime during this endocrine conflict, the perimenopause makes its appearance.

Depending largely upon the rate of ovarian decline, the perimenopause begins to be felt in the early forties, although women with exceedingly active and healthy ovaries may not experience the PeriMPX until their middle or late forties. Whenever it occurs, it precedes the menopause by two or three years and flows directly into it.

One of the most noticeable changes of the perimenopause involves menstruation. Because progesterone is no longer being secreted, the menstrual flow is liable to be considerably different. Estrogen alone cannot produce a normal endometrium capable of producing a normal period. Bleeding will, in some way, be different during the PeriMPX. Such alterations may be minor—bleeding may be slightly more irregular, somewhat shorter, or somewhat longer—and sometimes prolonged and heavy periods may be the order of the day.

Although bleeding irregularities and problems may arise in the PeriMPX as it leads into the MPX, a number of women have noted that menstruation can cease abruptly with no prior warnings. And unless hormone replacement is instituted, these women never menstruate again. Yet no matter what the pattern, the perimenopause usually involves some menstrual change.

SYMPTOMS OF THE PERIMENOPAUSE

Vague symptoms may appear at the start of the PeriMPX, signaling the beginning of ovarian failure. Fatigue, which is recorded in 75 percent of all women at this time, is probably the commonest companion of the perimenopause. Although fatigue is a symptom of many other disorders, its almost unfailing appearance is a common characteristic of the PeriMPX.

Emotional changes—particularly if PMS problems have been present—accelerate at this time. Insomnia (which may contribute to fatigue), depression (which may do the same thing), and irritability are common pitfalls. All of these symptoms, including fatigue, are variable and intermittent. They come and go and are not necessarily cyclic or related to the menstrual cycle.

THE DIAGNOSIS OF THE PERIMENOPAUSE

There is no known diagnostic sign to assist with the identification of the PeriMPX. Although blood FSH levels may be elevated, they bear no relationship to the symptoms of the PeriMPX. The levels of estrogen and progesterone change so imperceptibly that their measurement is of no use (until progesterone disappears altogether as ovulation ceases). The sensitivity of organs targeted by estrogen and progesterone—the uterus, the breasts, the skin, and the vagina—changes as well, but again the change is too slight to be of use in diagnosis. Insidious changes also begin to take place in bone density and in the blood vessels, but these changes occur without symptoms and are almost impossible to measure clinically.

It is clear, and has been said many times before, that not *all* women need or want any help at this time. Minimal or nonexistent symptoms require no supportive therapy by physicians. Nevertheless, regular gynecological examinations and consultations are important for all perimenopausal women, symptoms or not. Seemingly trifling problems that may arise at this time can, if neglected, ignite into crippling disorders in later years.

Annual or semiannual examinations and consultations are the cornerstone of proper PeriMPX management. The frequency of these visits depends upon your level of symptoms and complications.

Examinations should be preceded by a problem-oriented consultation. Such talks should be conducted with both participants sitting up. This has not always been so—as many of you already know. Modern examining equipment and enlightened competitive gynecologists, however, have largely dispelled the unequal environment.

You should have a Papanicolaou (Pap) smear done at least once a year, whether or not a hysterectomy has previously been performed. (See page 54.) Your doctor should take your blood pressure, record your height and weight, and do a urinalysis and a blood count.

Less frequent, but equally important, are tests of the blood fats—cholesterol, triglycerides, and others—plus regular mammograms and a baseline one-time bone density test. A hormone smear is also recommended.

THE TREATMENT OF THE PERIMENOPAUSE

Your postexamination consultation should include a discussion of any positive findings and help reinforce the significant aspects of your lifestyle—diet and exercise, along with drug, nicotine, and alcohol control. In addition, you should discuss the possible need for calcium and vitamin D supplements as well as for hormone replacement therapy.

If sufficient abnormal bleeding or subjective symptoms are present and HRT is indicated, certain oral contraceptives are perfect for the job. Here are some things about the oral contraceptive pill, or OC, that you might want to know:

• OCs cannot be used under any circumstances for women who smoke. A women who is addicted to tobacco at this time in her life subjects herself to a tenfold increase in death from heart disease if she uses OCs. Most nonsmokers may, however, use OCs with safety. The pill will resolve the nonsmoker's perimenopausal problems and keep her from conceiving (pregnancy is a condition that, at this time of a woman's life, involves much much greater risks than does the pill).

• Oral contraceptives do not increase the risk of gallbladder disease. Instead, they offer protection against certain pelvic infections and may also protect against anemia from excessive menstrual blood loss.

• There is increasing evidence that OCs protect the breasts, the ovaries, and the lining of the uterus from cancer, even for years after the OCs have been discontinued.

For these and other reasons, the birth control pill may be an ideal agent in managing the perimenopause. Some general medical problems (high blood pressure, for instance) may mitigate this fact. Your gynecologist will best advise you.

Because all the topics covered in a physical examination and consultation are so very important, they will be discussed in greater detail in the chapters that follow.

❧ *Pause and Reflect*

According to the Census Bureau in Washington, there will be 6.2 billion people on earth by the year 2000. In comparison, there were 3 billion in 1960. Although the United States population will not reproduce as rapidly as that of some Third World countries, there will still be a hefty increase in our population—at a rate of four every second!

Our population mix will change considerably by this century's end. Today's yuppies will be senior citizens by then. The menopausal population will be vastly larger and will continue to be a enlightened coterie with money to burn and the good sense not to burn it.

Another interesting explosion is taking place. Over 6,000 medical articles see print every day. Every day! Right now the body of our scientific information *doubles* every five years, and will soon double every two years. How much of that do you think your doctor can read?

Precious little—and work at the same time. Your doctor has to be helped by computer and other summary services to digest what new information is important to her.

And while we are on the subject of gynecologists—and women—it has been proven that female physicians spend more time with their patients than do their male counterparts. Moreover, in 1986 there were, for the first time, more female than male residents specializing in obstetrics and gynecology. Not only that, the pass rate for certification examination in obstetrics and gynecology was greater for females than males.

In addition, women believe their gynecologists are more honest than anyone other than members of the clergy! More honest than their own husbands! Least honest? Auto mechanics (17%), the President (8%), and Congress (3%).

Women outlive men, but this fact may soon change. Men are not getting healthier; women are catching more of men's problems. Why? Women are increasingly beset by high blood pressure, obesity and diabetes; the incidence of lung cancer in women has risen *600 percent* in the past thirty years, and lung cancer now kills more women than men; more women are involved with alcohol and drugs, as well as with cigarettes, because of changing societal roles and stresses; more women now suffer from suicidal depression; and breast cancer strikes one woman in eleven. The greatest insult among all these is smoking.

CHAPTER FOUR

The Menopause

The vagaries of semantics are nowhere more obvious than with the word "menopause." As already noted in the first chapter, the menopause (MPX) signifies, scientifically, *only the absolute cessation of menses.* At least, that is the present-day definition of the menopause. Yet the word "menopause," as it is popularly used, signifies the whole panorama of events and symptoms that flow from the onset of the MPX and encompasses all that happens in the ensuing several years—both physical and emotional. This includes not only the cessation of periods but the starting of the "change"—of flushes and sweats and insomnia and fatigue and all the other events that may be waiting in the wings.

But the proper word for this continuum of insults is the *climacteric.* Scientists, gynecologists, endocrinologists, and everyone else involved in menopausal management use this word to describe all the events that we are talking about and that you are struggling with. In fact, the leading clinics for the treatment of "the change of life" and what follows are called

"Climacteric Clinics." I tried to start a clinic using that name but only people with sexual problems came to see me, so I had to rename it.

These definitions are clearly established in medical literature. You and I, however, will continue to call all the things that are happening at the time of your life when menstruation ceases and *shortly* thereafter "the menopause (MPX)," and will call those things that follow these tumultuous events and last forever "the postmenopause (PMPX)."

Our final definition of the menopause, then, is the cessation of natural menstruation and the events (symptoms) that shortly precede and follow it.

Having resolved the issue of terms—at least to our satisfaction—it is safe to move on.

Moving on is what the menopause is all about. You are already aware that those things that are happening when menstruation ceases *do not* represent an abrupt change in function or a sudden decline in body function.

Slowly, but inexorably, ovarian function continues to subside as certain landmark events take place. As we noted earlier, ovulation ceases and with it, the production and secretion of progesterone. Estrogen secretion from the ovaries declines gradually until not enough is produced to support and bring forth a menstrual flow.

It is clear that if the ovaries have been surgically removed or if ovarian function has been destroyed by disease, there follows an abrupt and complete cessation of both estrogen and progesterone production. This event may evoke profound bodily changes that we will also look at as we move along.

Let's note here that the ovaries will continue to make *some* estrogen and estrogen-like substances, probably throughout your entire life, although this is a variable phenomenon. Many estrogen-like substances that the ovary produces at this time have masculinizing elements in their structure. Such elements may account for an increase in sex drive in certain postmenopausal women and for certain masculinizing tendencies, such as an increase in facial hair, that these women may exhibit.

There are two basic ovarian estrogens: estrone (E1) and estradiol (E2).

The production of E1 and E2 parallel one another during normal menstrual life as they are both excreted by maturing follicles. E2 is a more powerful estrogen than E1. Before the menopause, a small amount of E1 is made from a circulating male-like hormone called androstenedione. This conversion takes place in fatty tissues. After the menopause, more androstenedione (95 percent of which is made in the adrenal gland and 5 percent of which is produced in the ovaries) is converted to E1 in fatty tissue. This fact accounts for *some* of the postmenopause estrogen in heavy women. Moreover, increasing postmenopausal dominance of androstenedione produces masculine-like tendencies in some older women—facial hair growth and breast atrophy—and even increased sex drive.

Since E2 is primarily the product of the developing follicle, its levels drops dramatically at the menopause. Thereafter it is produced in small amounts by conversion of E1 in target organs such as the breasts.

You will see as our story unfolds on how these variable hormone factors can affect the outcome of the menopausal treatment.

When Does the Menopause Occur?

We have already noted that menstruation may cease when a woman is anywhere between forty-five and fifty years of age. This has been historically true. In addition:

• There are ethnic variations in menopausal onset but the studies reporting such differences are poorly controlled for other variables such as health, nutrition, and climate.

• Neither the age at which menstruation begins nor family history have any influence on the time of menopause.

• Thin women, malnourished women and women who smoke all have a significantly earlier menopause.

• The effect of marital status and family size upon entry into menopause is hotly debated and unsettled. A single recent study indicates that women who have sustained repeated abortions may have an earlier menopause.

• Higher altitudes produce an earlier menopause.

• The effect of long-term birth control pill usage upon menopausal onset is, as yet, unknown.

What Is the Menopause Like?

The menopause is comprised of many symptoms. Not every woman experiences all of them, and not all symptoms are felt with equal depth. Thus flushes may be incapacitating to some, but only minor nuisances to others. Listed below are the major symptoms associated with the menopause.

HOT FLASHES (FLUSHES) AND NIGHT SWEATS

Typically a flush starts deep within the chest, as intense heat, and flows upward and outward through the shoulders, neck and head. It is followed by some degree of sweating. The sufferer feels this heat and is aware, rightly or wrongly, that everyone can see the flush. Such episodes end in a few moments and can recur every few minutes or hours, depending upon a number of circumstances. Often, there follows a short period of faintness or weakness.

Here, with some simplification, is the actual sequence of physiological events in a typical hot flush cycle. Diminished estrogen levels irritate certain sensitive neurorceptors in the base of the brain. These neuroreceptors in turn signal peripheral blood vessels in the upper body to dilate (expand). We are now just a few minutes away from a flush.

Gradually the dilated blood vessels heat up the skin and as that happens, a flush unfolds. While skin temperature is rising during the several minutes of a flush, body core temperature begins to drop a few degrees. This cooling effect is heightened because newly formed perspiration evaporates from the skin. Chills may now follow this double cooling phenomenon.

As a result of body cooling, the hormone adrenalin begins to circulate; the adrenal gland is invoking its "involuntary fight or flight" response. Peripheral blood vessels constrict and the flush ends. Five minutes have elapsed.

Some other things happen during a flush. Oxygen consumption increases. So does the pulse rate. Electrocardiograph recordings reveal fluctuations in heartbeat outside normal limits, but clearly without harmful effect.

Although flushes are the most common symptom of the menopause, their intensity and occurrence rate varies greatly from one woman to another. Nevertheless, 85 percent of all menopausal women experience flushes for over a year and up to 50 percent for over five years.

Night sweats are essentially the same as the daytime flushing phenomenon, but work their magic during normal sleep. Heat generated by the flush that occurs while you are sleeping makes you kick off your sheets and blankets; this subconscious baring of the flesh is naturally followed by body coolness from evaporating sweat. Thus the classic nocturnal "cold sweat."

External stimuli can initiate a hot flush. Thus, a doorbell ring, a sudden auto stop, a phone call from your gynecologist, a new perfume scent—any number of things can "turn up the heat." Dreams can also cause night sweats.

Unlike many of the serious long-term consequences of the MPX (osteoporosis, for instance), flushes and sweats gradually diminish and disappear after a variable number of years. Hormone replacement therapy completely obliterates flushes and sweats.

INSOMNIA

"Think in the morning. Act in the noon. Eat in the evening. Sleep in the night."

Good advice for all times, but sleep may be denied those of you struggling with the menopause. Insomnia becomes a companion almost as faithful as flushes. And there are several reasons why this is so.

A hot flush brings wakefulness, and the cold sweat that follows each flush requires the readjustment of sheets, covers, coverlets, quilts, pillows and your bedfellow. And when that's all over with, you're about 10,000 behind on the sheep count. Even if sleep comes again, there is another night sweat waiting close by in the wings. And it all starts again.

Depression is clearly associated with the menopause and it involves a significant number of menopausal women. Since early-morning wakefulness is a common companion of depression it may therefore involve MPX women, even when night sweats do not.

Other menopausal associates—irritability, heart palpitations and formications (numb, itchy or irritable extremities)—can all contribute to restless nights.

Clearly, there is an abundance of reasons why you should not sleep well during the MPX—and the lack of sound, uninterrupted sleep probably contributes heavily to fatigue. Fortunately, hormone replacement therapy will control almost all menopausal insomnia.

FATIGUE

Every once in a while a patient of long standing will arrive for her annual visit and consultation complaining of "fatigue."

Now in her early forties, my patient friend will still have regular periods, no hot flushes or night sweats, excellent health and habits, will sleep well and have no family or work problems, but will be inexplicably exhausted. She gets up in limbo, drags during the day and is ready for the sheets before the Cosby show is over.

Generally, a complete physical examination and the standard blood work will yield no helpful information. And that is because her "fatigue" is really one of the earliest indications of the MPX, which, as we already know, may be first noted in the perimenopause.

It is important here for the patient and the physician to be certain that there are no physical or emotional causes for the tiredness other than the menopause itself. Sleep must be adequate, sustained and relatively free from interruptions. In addition, nighttime visits to the bathroom need to be recorded since they tend to become more of a constant presence at this time and signal the beginnings of the menopause.

EMOTIONAL PROBLEMS

Scientists and physicians—both male and female—who have studied the menopause as a career cannot agree upon the psychological content of the menopause and, in many cases, simply state their own convictions. Gynecologists have just now begrudgingly added emotional problems to their lexicon of menopausal symptoms.

No matter what the opinions are or who holds them, one thing has been clearly proven: hormone replacement therapy will alleviate menopausal emotional problems.

Here is a list of the commonest emotional symptoms found in the menopause: depression, irritability, anxiety, insomnia, tension, antisocial behavior, headaches, inability to concentrate, loss of sex drive, nervousness, aggressiveness.

Over half of all menopausal women will experience some (but not all) of these disturbances, and they may last for several years. It is important that they be differentiated from the true psychological illnesses that might well occur coincidentally at this time. Thus a depression may be MPX-related or may be a true and separate entity requiring special treatment. Clearly, such unrelated depressions do not respond to hormone therapy. The same is true of other nonmenopausal-related psychological disorders.

SEXUALITY

As noted above, the desire for sexual activity often diminishes at this time. This timing may be coincidental since women's sexual appetite usually—but not always—begins to diminish slowly after the mid-thirties, and the change may become noticeable only in the mid-forties. Yet whatever the reason, loss of sexual drive is common during the menopause.

Other sexual changes become apparent as estrogen secretion diminishes. Erotic stimulation (local or general) fails to produce the usual vaginal lubrication. Time-to-orgasm may be increased, and orgasm may be difficult to achieve. Finally, as the vaginal skin becomes thinner and drier, intercourse becomes more painful and vaginal infections more common.

These changes do not take place instantly at the menopause. They are gradual events that increase in intensity over several years. Women who, somehow, somewhere, continue to make limited amounts of estrogen may exhibit few of these sexual changes until very late in their postmenopausal years. And certain women, because of the increase of male-like hormones in their postmenopausal life, will experience an increase in sexual drive.

The effect of hormone replacement on sexual drive is very complex and will be looked at carefully later on. (See pages 112–14.)

LESS COMMON MENOPAUSE PROBLEMS

FORMICATIONS. This questionable-sounding word designates conditions that affect the skin and peripheral tissues. Itchy, numb, tingling arms and legs, fidgety feet, tender joints and so forth are included in this category.

PALPITATIONS. When you become consciously aware of your heartbeat, whether it's fast, slow or irregular, you are experiencing palpitations. Palpitations are generally accompanied by feelings of apprehension and anxiety, but when palpitations are a symptom of the menopause, the condition does not signify harm.

There are other disorders that will produce palpitations—at any time of life—and care must be taken in assigning this symptom to the menopause. On the other hand, simple menopausal palpitations are frequently and falsely diagnosed as heart disorders; both doctors and patients must be aware of this symptom of the menopause and treat it accordingly.

LOSS OF MEMORY (FOR RECENT EVENTS ONLY). You remember your third cousin's birthday but can't remember where you set your drink down. Or you can remember your 1968 income tax payment but can't remember why you just got in the car. Some physicians say that such memory loss comes from an inability to concentrate, but whatever the cause, it is real and it is a nuisance.

ONGOING PROBLEMS

It is important to remember that other events that we have already alluded to continue their march through the menopausal territory. Because of estrogen depletion, bone loss accelerates, arteriosclerosis accelerates, fertility declines and disappears, sexual organs atrophy, and skin and breast tissue lose tone and elasticity. These problems will be mentioned again in great detail in our discussion of the postmenopause for, although they start here, they continue to work their will in the years that follow.

How Is the Menopause Diagnosed?

With all these symptoms occurring to one degree or another, what signs are present to help physicians make the diagnosis of menopause? Not many.

After taking the menopausal history, your doctor will proceed to examine you (the components of this exam will be outlined in the next chapter). Such a physical examination reveals few of the vast changes that slowly brought you to the menopause. Everything appears the same as it did one year ago—or five years ago (unless you have some other problems— like excess weight or high blood pressure—that has overtaken you).

What about lab tests? The only procedure of real diagnostic help is a test for an elevated blood FSH level. This hormone, you recall, is secreted by the pituitary gland during reproductive life to stimulate ovarian activity. As the ovary continues to fail, the pituitary sends out more FSH to try to revive the ovary. Of course, the FSH is useless as the ovarian decline is relentless and irreversible. But FSH elevation is positive proof of the menopausal presence.

Vaginal hormone smears have been used extensively to measure body estrogen levels and to follow hormone therapy programs. But such smears, while easy to take and read, are not accurate enough to confirm early onset of the meno-pause—only the advanced menopause—or the results of hor-mone therapy.

So we are left with little to help us confirm the diagnosis of menopause save the patient's symptoms and the absence of menses. *And that's plenty.* The symptoms and the absence of menses signify the onset of the menopause. From here we continue our journey into the issues you face in your menopau-sal years.

◄§ *Pause and Reflect*

The following facts about estrogen and flushes indicate that hot flashes occur *only* following estrogen withdrawal:

• Women born with congenitally nonfunctional ovaries—thus never making estrogen—also never have hot flashes. Similarly, girls who lose their ovaries because of some catas-trophe (like early ovarian malignancy) before menstruation even begins also never have hot flashes.

• Men who have been treated for cancer of the prostate gland with estrogen will have hot flashes when the estrogen is discontinued.

Other problems may produce flush-like episodes:

• People with vasomotor instability blush a lot and have fainting spells at the drop of a thermostat. It is a lifelong characteristic, however.

• High blood pressure, especially when out of control, can often cause recurrent facial flushes. Affecting both men and women, the flushes disappear with appropriate hypertension therapy.

• An overactive (hyperactive) thyroid will often cause flushes which, again, disappear when the thyroid comes under control.

• Emotional problems, including panic attacks, anxiety and depression, also cause flushes.

Do women in other cultures experience the same symptoms at the menopause? The answer to that question is difficult to give because of language barriers, cultural differences and bias on the part of investigators—to name a few of the study problems. Nevertheless, here are some findings:

• 482 Rajput women living in India reported that the menopause was a welcome event noted only because of menstrual cessation. The absence of menstrual flow signaled an incredible elevation of stature for these women. Women were released from a veiled, secluded life in a compound to talk and socialize (even drink) with menfolk. They then became revered as models of wisdom and experience by the younger generation.

• According to one study, Zulu women noted little menopausal symptomology. Another study of Zulu women, however, revealed that many had menopausal problems similar to women in Western societies. Different investigators.

• In all studies of menopausal symptoms, regardless of race, creed, color, social or economic status, one fact stands out: Women who are well-integrated in their environment, who are surrounded by friends, and who possess a good social network and have meaningful activities will have less intense menopausal symptoms.

―――――――

When scientists first suggested using sex hormones for the treatment of depression (in both sexes), they were hooted out of scientific circles, even though the premise was supported by excellent research. Forty years later, however, the data has been "rediscovered," and, indeed, sex hormones now have a valid place in the treatment of many depressions.

―――――――

If you believe in teleology (the study of final causes, or the philosophy that things have a purposeful end) then you can believe that nature has provided women with a hormonal edge that protects them during the reproductive years. A woman is more resilient to stress and is protected against the harmful consequences of a high-fat diet as long as she has estrogen. When reproduction is beyond her capabilities, her risk of cardiovascular disease matches that of men.

CHAPTER FIVE

How to Survive—
and Even Enjoy—
the Menopause

Getting through a childhood could be a very deadly game, were it not for some human contrivances. Vaccines, antibiotics, surgical interventions, burn therapies, leukemia treatment, pasteurized milk, seat harness laws, and many more human contrivances have helped to make passage through childhood safe.

So it is with the menopause. Safe and positive passage requires some human contrivances and some human intervention. Listed below are the interventions that are important for you.

Medical Care

Your primary care physician should be a gynecologist. There are three classes of gynecologists, namely:

• *Generalists.* This category includes gynecologists who conduct a general gynecology practice doing routine female surgical procedures. These physicians also often continue to practice obstetrics.

• *Gynecological oncologists.* These doctors restrict their practice to the management of malignant disorders of the female organs.

• *Infertility gynecologists.* As the name implies, sterility and infertility is the field of interest that engages these gynecologists.

You want a general gynecologist to manage your menopause. The doctors in the other two categories are trying desperately to keep up with their own specialty fields of interest, and as a result they are not as well-versed in the management of the menopause. (Be aware that not all general gynecologists will be interested in treating the menopause; make sure your gynecologist's goals coincide with yours.)

While it is true that almost all physicians can do a routine pelvic, Pap smear and breast examination, it is equally true that hormone replacement therapy has become so complicated that not even all gynecologists are interested in tackling it.

Therefore, I recommend that you seek the care of a competent, caring gynecologist who is interested in menopausal management. There are plenty of them around. If you live in a community that does not have a gynecologist, your own family physician will manage your menopause, checking any problems with a consultant gynecologist as he or she feels necessary.

A successful relationship with your physician requires bilateral openness and willingness to trot out problems on both sides of the desk—or whatever device your consultation takes place over. You, for instance, have to feel free to say that your vagina doesn't lubricate during sex like in the good old days, and your doctor has to feel free to ask you whether your vagina lubricates during sex like it did in the good old days. It is fundamental to your proper care that you tell all you know to be wrong—even if your doctor does not have the good sense to ask for it. Drop at least five of your seven veils.

Since your commitment to your doctor (and your doctor's commitment to you) should be a lengthy one—and hopefully one that has preceded the menopause by some years—you might want to consider your *responsibilities to each other* from now on. Here, for what it's worth, are some of my views.

THE DOCTOR

Listed below are your doctor's responsibilities. He or she should

• Ensure adequate examinations and testing at your regular visits. Arrange for out-of-office examinations (mammograms, blood work, etc.). Properly chart and accumulate data generated by tests and examinations.

• Provide information—with your written permission—to other physicians as you request it, and withhold personal information from all others. Please note that, even if you're not aware of it, you have surrendered this right to privacy to your insurance company and to anyone with whom they wish to share information. That may include other insurance companies, the Federal Government and your employer's insurance clerk. That's worth remembering.

• Completely disclose benefits and risks when giving—or denying—a certain medication program. "Complete" disclosure means a lot of things. If your doctor suggests surgery at some point, the major risks and benefits need to be laid out for you (although it is impossible to explore every potential risk and benefit). The same is true when discussing hormone replacement therapy.

• Be reasonably available and reasonably current in the areas of his or her responsibility.

• Cover general health problems with you. As doctors, we are very inadequate in this regard. Studies show that we often fail to discuss the elimination of tobacco, moderation of alcohol, use of seat belts, importance of good exercise and dietary habits—the list could go on and on. These things will hurt more of you than the things doctors spend hours talking about. We are as guilty of neglecting to discuss these important health factors as you are of neglecting to practice them.

• Treat you with compassion and understanding. We physicians are healers—not judges, moralists or mechanics.

YOU

Listed below are your responsibilities. You should

• Keep your appointments and get scheduled tests taken care of as directed. Even if your physician does not send regular reminders through the mail or have his or her staff call you to set up routine visits, you must share some of the responsibility for keeping the relationship going. Somewhere you have a data bank of sorts where you store information and memos. Punch it in.

• Ask questions when you are uncertain about a proposed treatment or procedure or if you don't understand the information you have been given.

• Get a second opinion when you are in real doubt about a proposed therapy plan—be it in surgery, hormone replacement, or thermal baths—or about anything your doctor suggests which is major in scope and with which you do not generally agree. Most of the time, your doctor will welcome a second opinion, for it usually will confirm his or her position and strengthen your relationship. Also, remember *your* doctor is *someone else's* second opinion. Think about that.

• Comply with your doctor's recommendations. Compliance is one of your major responsibilities. It's yours alone because you have to do the complying. Studies show that, with the possible exception of birth control pills, only about one-third of all clients or patients continue to follow advice or take medications. So follow the dietary, exercise and other general health measures with which you are provided. It's your doctor's responsibility to give such advice. In addition, take medications exactly as outlined, in the amount and at the times prescribed. More is not better and your friend's medicine is probably not right for you. If your medication disagrees with you in any real way, call your doctor.

We have, of course, outlined a perfect doctor/patient relationship—one that exists only between a perfect doctor and a perfect patient in a perfect world. Since that is not the way things are, we must make the best of what we have.

MEDICAL VISITS

How often should you visit your gynecologist? Every 6 to 12 months, if there are no complications requiring closer attention.

What is accomplished at this visit? Following a discussion of present symptoms, a regular examination is performed, including a breast and pelvic examination and the measurement of weight, height and blood pressure. In addition, laboratory work is done that includes a Pap smear, urine and blood count, and perhaps a hormone smear.

When indicated, a mammogram, a bone density, and detailed blood tests may be arranged. Also, a more detailed physical examination may be called for if unusual symptoms are present.

These, in general, are the same procedures that we outlined in the management of the perimenopause. The consultation that follows at this time will, however, deal more specifically with hormone replacement and its management.

Here are some common medical terms that you should know:

PAP SMEAR. This test is named after the Greek-born American anatomist Papanicolaou, who discovered it and persuaded doctors the world over to use it to detect cancer. This smear is taken from the cervix, which is a common site for cancer. The Pap smear can almost always detect the presence of cells destined to cause cancer of the cervix in the future. The smear is of value *only* in screening for malignant and premalignant changes on the cervix or, more rarely, the back of the vagina.

HORMONE SMEAR. Also known as the *maturation index,* this smear, taken from the vaginal wall, can roughly determine estrogen levels within the body. This is based on the fact that only estrogen can cause the vaginal lining to mature, and thus this amount of estrogen mirrors the levels of estrogen are circulating within the body. Estrogen given vaginally as a cream or suppository will, of course, produce a false reading because of its local activity.

BLOOD PROFILES. With automated chemistry, doctors can now easily and relatively cheaply obtain a profile of many body organ systems with one sample of blood. Also known as a *SMAC profile*, a blood profile measures liver and kidney function, blood lipids (or fats, such as cholesterol and triglycerides), sugar, enzymes, electrolytes, thyroid function, serum iron, blood count, and often more. Such chemical tests are often important in careful management of the menopause.

Caring for Yourself

While regular contact with your physician is vitally important, there are other things to be done at this time that are also necessary in managing your menopause. Your physician should review much of this substantial material with you at regular visits, and reinforce it from time to time. If your doctor fails to do so, you can learn about it here, even though your own doctor is your best source of information and help.

DIET

Of course, what you eat has been, is now, and will always be of vital importance to you and your well-being.

We are concerned not only with how much we eat but with what we eat. Certain culinary truths prevail:

- We need *fewer* and *fewer* calories per day each year of our lives from now on. "I don't eat any more than I ever did but I still gain!" is a cop-out.

- Too much of our diet is fat.

- Weight is a variable depending entirely on what we consume and how much of it is burned as energy.

• Some people can eat more than others and still not gain weight. Conversely, some people can eat less than others and still gain weight.

It is important to follow a diet that is low in fat and one that will not provide you more calories than you need. There are many diet principles that you need to follow; refer to Chapter 6 for a complete discussion of healthful eating. It is an important part of your menopausal and postmenopausal life.

EXERCISE

It is mind-boggling to contemplate all the devices, the spas, the aerobic classes, the Marquis de Sade running clubs and all the other forced-labor camps that have sprung up to compensate for the physical inactivity that the good life has brought us. The truth is, walking, swimming, cycling or *light*-impact aerobics is all anyone needs.

Exercise is important for cardiovascular fitness and the maintenance of bone strength. It should be regular, enjoyable and productive, though you must be careful not to overexert yourself, as excess exercise can cause damage. Again, a whole section is devoted to proper exercise programs, starting on page 84.

HABITS

Our personal habits—as we have been told so many times— are the chains that bind us. Some of our habits are good, and some are bad. Usually a lot are bad. The bad ones have a way of intruding upon the menopause and must be set aside.

Habits that revolve around sleep and hygiene, nicotine, alcohol and drugs, travel, hobbies and sports, and more may have to be revised. Some even dropped. Pages 86–92 refer to these issues in greater detail.

SEX

From what you already understand about the hormonal, physical and emotional changes that are taking place at the menopause, it is clear that the sexual drives and gratifications are in for some sort of upheaval, or at least a regrouping. These new experiences and the physical changes that accompany them need not lead to sexual frustration and disharmony; they can actually lead to a more fulfilled and rewarding sexual life. More about that too, in Chapter 7.

Hormone Replacement Therapy

This is the centerpiece of MPX management. Most gynecologists now feel that hormone replacement therapy should be offered to every menopausal woman who has no insurmountable contraindication. The present methods of administration have been proven to be so safe and so effective that there is really little argument remaining against its regular use.

HRT has had a history filled with controversy. Both estrogen and progesterone equivalents were available for clinical use by the end of World War II. Progesterone was perceived to be of no value in managing the menopause since it offered no relief for any recognized menopausal problem. Estrogen, on the other hand, provided prompt and unmatched relief. Indeed, flushes and sweats, along with a variety of emotional problems, completely vanished as estrogen levels rose. (At that time, these urgent symptoms were the major recognized menopausal assaults, and the ones that needed to be treated.)

Accordingly, estrogen therapy for the menopause became very much in vogue. The hormone was widely given—often in unusually large doses—and for a while, women found relief from the unpleasant symptoms of the menopause.

But before long, snags began to appear in the forever-estrogen fabric. Cases of excessive uterine bleeding and of intravascular clotting (thrombosis) were reported in the literature in increasing numbers. Most devastating of all, an increased harvest of uterine (specifically, endometrial) cancer became a clear component of unilateral, prolonged estrogen administration.

Thus, by 1970, estrogen treatment of the menopause had fallen by the wayside, a victim not only of abuse but of unacceptable consequences.

During the decade that followed, significant clinical research involving the use of progesterone to allay the chronic irritative aspects of unopposed estrogen yielded good news. It was demonstrated, to almost universal agreement, that an estrogen-progesterone combination not only represented a safe menopausal treatment, but also actually appeared to protect the patient from uterine cancer, breast cancer, and, perhaps, certain other problems.

Thus, the modern hormone replacement therapy program was born. Modern HRT almost always includes various *combinations* of *estrogen* and *progesterone,* although there is still some difference of opinion about the addition of progesterone after a hysterectomy has been performed. Moreover, the male hormone testosterone is now being used in certain circumstances. And that brings up the subject of HRT risks and benefits.

HRT RISKS

What are the risks of HRT?

• Estrogen may, by its effect on liver metabolism and function, increase the risk of high blood pressure, gallstones, and intravascular clotting. *Oral* estrogen is more likely to do this since it is absorbed via the digestive system and must pass through the liver before entering the general circulation. Abnormal liver function, however, is unusual with modern estrogen dosage levels.

• High dosages of estrogens can and do alter sugar metabolism adversely. However, this usually occurs with higher dosages (birth control pills, for example) than with dosages used in the menopause. In fact, HRT is generally not contraindicated for women with diabetes. No long-term studies of the effect of *combined* estrogen-progesterones on carbohydrate metabolism have yet been completed.

• There is a clear, firm and deadly relationship between smoking and the use of birth control pills. The combination—particularly in women past the age of thirty-five—increases the risk of heart attacks by an astounding rate. Oral HRT *may* have the same deadly connection and is usually not prescribed for heavy smokers. Non-oral routes may be safer, but even this is not yet clearly established.

• Estrogen usually increases the level of high-density lipoproteins (HDL) in the blood. (See pages 82–84.) This is altogether good, as it reduces the risks of heart disease. However, progesterone compounds have been shown to decrease this beneficial effect. So we have an apparent standoff.

• If you are still fertile, can you get pregnant on HRT? Yes, you can. You can also win the Publishers Clearing House sweepstakes. Your chances are about the same in either event. But check this carefully with your doctor. Pregnancy, of course, is an *absolute* contraindication to HRT.

• Certain disorders of the reproductive organs prevent or limit the use of HRT. And HRT may nourish these problems.

Fibroid uterine tumors (myomata), very common benign growths that appear singly or in clusters on and in the uterine muscle, appear to be nourished and to grow in the presence of estrogen. They must be watched carefully if HRT is to be administered.

Endometriosis is another common gynecological problem that is certainly dependent upon estrogen for survival. In this condition, which may arise when a woman is in her thirties, blood-filled cysts begin to appear on and around the uterus, tubes and ovaries and produce significant pelvic pain as they grow. Under the microscope the cysts appear identical to the endometrium that is normally found lining the uterine cavity. Endometriosis must be destroyed before HRT may be considered.

Cancer of the endometrium very definitely contraindicates HRT. Although the vast majority of present-day literature supports the claim that modern HRT does not cause this highly curable cancer, nevertheless estrogen will certainly nourish such a growth. Thus it must be removed before HRT can be considered. More about that later.

Testosterone therapy may induce facial hair growth and deepening of the voice and must be closely monitored.

Now, to the good news.

HRT BENEFITS

What are the benefits of HRT?

• Control of menopausal symptoms.

• Control of osteoporosis.

• Delay of arteriosclerosis and the attendant heart disease.

• Protection of the sexual life.

• Long-term studies indicate that the risk of endometrial and breast cancer appear to be actually reduced among women on a combined (estrogen-progesterone) HRT program.

That is certainly enough to make it all worthwhile.

Principles of HRT Administration

WHEN TO START

Although some gynecologists prefer to wait until the MPX is well established (perhaps a year after the menses cease) before starting HRT, logic does not support such a stand. Significant discomfort and irreparable system damage may take place during that time. And nothing is gained.

Accordingly, most of us begin HRT during the PeriMPX, particularly since new evidence indicates that loss of bone mass may begin well before the cessation of menses (see Chapter 9).

Certain studies must precede HRT:

• A complete gynecological examination, including a Pap smear.

• A screening mammogram that shows no evidence of suspicious breast changes.

• In some cases, laboratory blood analysis for blood lipids (cholesterols and triglycerides) may be indicated.

HOW HRT IS GIVEN

Estrogen may be given in five ways:

• *Oral pills.* Both estrone and estradiol may be taken by mouth. Estrone (Premarin, Ogen and other brands) is the most popular oral estrogen, but estradiol (Estinyl, for instance) is gaining in popularity. Both are effective and generally well-tolerated. For a variety of reasons (headaches and digestive irritation and swelling are the commonest reasons; read your package inserts), some women are unable to take oral estrogen. And in some rare cases, oral estrogens appear to be ineffective and useless.

• *Intramuscular injections.* Both estrone and estradiol may be given by injection. Estradiol in oil is most commonly used since it is absorbed slowly and needs be given only at 2- to 4-week intervals. Injected estrogen goes directly into the circulation without first passing through the liver. This has both good and bad effects, as we have seen. The main drawbacks of intramuscular injections, however, are the discomfort of regular injections plus the peaks and valleys of estrogen levels that such a system inevitably produces.

• *Transdermal patches.* Recently introduced in this country, estradiol reservoirs that stick to the skin and release regular amounts of estrogen *transdermally* (across the skin) have become enormously in vogue. The patches are worn constantly (below the waist and, by many women, on the buttocks and flanks) and are changed twice weekly. Their distinct advantage is a relatively constant and even flow of estrogen into the body day and night, with no peaks or valleys and, thus, fewer side effects related to over- or undersupply.

The estradiol in the patch is the same estradiol that is found in pills and shots, and the estrogen blood levels that can be attained by wearing the patches are the same as with oral and injectable administration; it is therefore possible that the patch achieves all the same benefits. (Although estradiol patches have not yet been proven effective against osteoporosis, it is only because they have not been around long enough to generate the necessary data.) As with shots, transdermal estradiol bypasses the liver. Also, it is now evident that the high-fiber diet recommended to all of us may wash out a portion of orally administered estrogen. The major problem with patches at this time is that a significant number of women develop skin irritation and may be forced to discontinue their use.

• *Subcutaneous pellets.* Usually inserted beneath the skin—*subcutaneously*—under a local anesthetic, pellets of estradiol have begun to have a following in this country after years of use abroad. Their duration of action is variable, but may be as long as 6 months. There are several problems inherent in this technique. In addition to the fact that the duration of action is variable, the pellets are difficult to remove should they prove disagreeable in any way. However, this technique is becoming more refined and more acceptable all the time.

• *Vaginal hormone creams.* For many, many years, vaginal applications of hormone creams have been used to treat postmenopausal vaginal changes. The creams have been used to reduce vaginal infections and painful sexual experiences. The beneficial effect was—and still is—often miraculous to the thin-skinned sufferer. It became clear early on that some of this vaginally applied estrogen was being absorbed into the body (it is absorbed by the same mechanisms as the modern patches). Thus some gynecologists used vaginal hormone creams and suppositories to achieve systemic effects. The method is not entirely esthetic and so is not often used today, however.

Progesterone is administered always as a *progestin* (also called a progestagen), which is a synthetic progesterone-like compound. Medroxyprogesterone (Provera) is used most commonly today, but there are others. Progestins are usually given by mouth in various combinations with estrogen. Injectable progestins are available, but rarely used in HRT. Finally, pure progesterone vaginal suppositories are becoming available in this country but they, too, are not commonly used in menopausal HRT (see the discussion of the premenstrual syndrome).

When a male hormone—testosterone—is indicated in HRT programs (see pages 112–14), it can be given in a number of ways:

• Oral tablets of testosterone may be given separately or combined with estrogen in fixed ratios. These tablets must, of course, go through the liver in their absorptive pass and thus lose some of their potency. There is, however, a sublingual testosterone tablet that, lodged under the tongue, releases the male hormone directly into the circulation.

• Injectable testosterone is available, with or without balancing amounts of estrogen.

• Testosterone pellets are now available for implantation under the skin in a manner similar to that used for estrogen pellets.

Male hormones are administered in certain HRT programs when sexual stimulation is indicated. Although testosterone is closely balanced with estrogen to prevent masculinizing side effects (excess hair growth, voice changes and clitoral enlargement, for example), the balance is not always perfect and so some of these side effects may occur. Most often they can be controlled by dosage changes.

HRT Programs

HRT is called for in several circumstances. Listed below are the circumstances and what is called for in each.

UTERUS AND OVARIES IN PLACE

The treatment program here, at this point in our scientific knowledge, causes the menstrual cycle and regular periods to continue for some time—until later in the postmenopausal life. This is not always welcome news, for some women hope to dispense with all unused tampons and pads. Techniques such as laser ablation (destruction) of the endometrium are under study now and eventually may allow HRT to be instituted without the continuation of menstruation, but for the time being, the menstrual cycle must continue regularly and normally. Thus the hormones must be taken in a cyclic manner much in the same way as birth control pills—to produce cyclic bleeding. Also, again we must be reasonably certain that there is no substantial pelvic disease, such as fibroids or endometriosis, that might be nourished by the estrogen replacement.

What are the methods of treatment in this case? There are four basic alternatives; they are described briefly below.

• Oral estrogen tablets are taken daily for 21 days. During the last 7 to 12 days, progestagen tablets are added to the program. Menstruation usually follows a few days after the last medication, and a new hormone cycle is begun on the fifth day of the flow. The dosages given vary somewhat dependent upon the physician's preferences and upon the responses of the patient. As the menopausal years go by, the hormone dosages and the combinations change, so that in women in their late fifties menses become but a trickle and may completely disappear. More on that when we discuss the postmenopause.

• Patches are generally used in a constant, uninterrupted manner—that is, two patches a week without cessation. In this program, progestagens are added orally for 7 to 12 days every fourth week. Menstruation is usually regulated in this manner, but menses are sometimes difficult to adjust with this relatively new approach. It is certainly worth the combined effort of patient and physician.

• Injectable hormones are usually given only if other HRT forms of treatment are, for one reason or another, unacceptable. Most often the hormones are suspended in oil so that they will be slowly absorbed, and thus need be given only twice in one cycle. The initial dose contains estrogen alone and is given on the fifth postmenstrual day. A second injection containing both estrogen and a progestagen is given 10 to 14 days later, depending upon the patient's menstrual response.

• Subcutaneous pellets are put in place as frequently as recurrent menopausal symptoms indicate—usually at 4- to 6-month intervals—and progestagens are given by mouth at 4-week intervals and for 10 to 12 days. Menstrual cycle adjustment may be difficult.

UTERUS REMOVED BUT OVARIES REMAIN

It may be several years after the uterus is removed (hysterectomy) before HRT therapy becomes necessary. It depends upon the woman's age at the time of surgery and upon the health of her ovaries. Thus, a woman who sustains a hysterectomy at thirty-five because of fibroids may not need to start HRT for ten years.

HRT is thus begun when menopausal symptoms appear, or when the vaginal hormone smear and/or the blood FSH indicate failing ovarian hormone production. In actual practice, the appearance of recognizable MPX symptoms (flushes and sweats, for instance) is all the evidence needed to establish a trial HRT program.

In the absence of the uterus there is no need to provide cyclic hormone replacement since there will be no bleeding. This is a great advantage.

There is no evidence that HRT has any effect, good or bad, upon the aging ovaries.

The plans, then, are as follows:

• Oral estrogen tablets are taken daily without any interruption or change in the dosage level.

• Transdermal estrogen continues unchanged, being replaced twice weekly.

• Injections continue to be given at 2-week intervals but often can be spaced somewhat farther apart.

• Subcutaneous pellets are replaced as often as necessary, at up to 6-month intervals.

Progestagens are not at this time widely used in HRT after the uterus is removed. Many gynecologists feel that, with the uterus gone, there is no longer any risk of cancer from unopposed estrogen. Other gynecologists (including this one) feel that progestagens are still very important because there is growing evidence that progestagens protect the breasts against cancer, and progestagens build *new* bone. Estrogen simply delays the destruction of *old* bone. (See the section on osteoporosis, Chapter 9.)

Accordingly, I feel that progestagens should still be given along with the constant estrogen program and in the same dosage range used in all the regular HRT programs.

UTERUS, TUBES AND OVARIES REMOVED

If the surgery removing the uterus, tubes and ovaries (hysterectomy and bilateral salpingo-oophorectomy) was for a cancer of the endometrium, hormone therapy may be absolutely contraindicated. (See below for further information.) If the surgery was for cancer of the cervix, HRT is not contraindicated. If the surgery was undertaken for the treatment of cancer of the ovaries, HRT must be decided upon on an individual basis.

Some gynecologists feel that HRT should not be used after this type of surgery if it was undertaken to remove extensive (or even early) endometriosis. That position, however, is not universally held, and many gynecologists begin hormone replacement therapy at once, in a modified way, usually employing large doses of progestagens or combining estrogen with the testosterone for the first few months. These programs must be tailored individually.

If there are no substantial contraindications to HRT, it should be started *immediately* after such surgery. The *younger* the patient, the *more important* this is.

The administration of HRT following this surgery is similar to that after an uncomplicated hysterectomy.

AFTER CANCER OF THE ENDOMETRIUM
OR OF THE BREASTS

It has always been considered incorrect to give HRT to a woman who has sustained a cancer of the endometrium or the breasts. After all, both tissues are estrogen targets in the first place, and estrogen, when given alone, has been found to cause cancer of the endometrium where none existed before. Furthermore, as many of you may know, most breast cancers are tested nowadays after removal for hormone dependency and many are estrogen-dependent or, estrogen targets, just like healthy breast tissue. For these and other reasons, leading experts have termed HRT ill-advised in such cancer cases, regardless of the severity of existing menopausal problems.

Recently, however, studies have begun to appear in which HRT has, in fact, been initiated in some women who have suffered these malignancies, provided

• At least five years have elapsed in which they have been free of any evidence of recurrence.

• Significant menopausal problems exist (osteoporosis, vaginal atrophy in young women, etc.)

• The patient requests it and is absolutely and completely informed of the known risks.

Although these programs are young and no hard and fast conclusions can as yet be drawn, HRT may become acceptable in such cases in the next few years. In this regard, there is recent evidence that proper HRT is safe to administer immediately after surgery for early (Stage I) cancer of the endometrium.

How Long Should HRT Last?

When, if ever, should hormone replacement cease? That depends to a large extent, upon which gynecologist you ask. This holds true whether the gynecologist is male or female. Remember, some don't think it is necessary at all, and some think it is only necessary for the first few years of the menopause, when bone loss is supposedly greatest and when symptoms are the worst. Finally, some believe you should take it as long as you live.

So we must go back to some of the basics. Your "menopause" only lasts a little while. The events that follow, however, last a long, long time. And so both of these things must be dealt with for a long, long time.

We have seen that the menopause represents an acute phase of ovarian decline and includes the cessation of monthly periods along with all the other symptoms—flushes, insomnia, fatigue, etc.—that surround it. Thereafter, there exists a hormone deficiency syndrome that induces or accelerates arteriosclerosis, osteoporosis, atrophic skin changes and multiple sexual dysfunctions in variable degrees. These are the postmenopausal years (PMPX). This is where you are going to spend the rest of your life, and most women find that HRT makes it all more enjoyable.

The Cost of HRT

Hormone costs vary from one part of the United States to another and in different parts of any one community. And if generics are substituted, the prices may be even more unpredictable.

Here are some sample prices as posted in a local chain drug store.

	BRAND NAME	GENERIC
Premarin (estrone) 1.25 mg	$30.98 per 100	$13.29 per 100
Estinyl (estradiol) .05 mg	$30.98 per 100	not available
Estraderm Patches (estradiol) .1 mg	$14.86 per 8	not available
Provera (progestagen or progestin) 10 mg	$24.69 per 50	$13.79 per 50
Delestrogen Injectable (estradiol) 20 mg/cc	$38.99 per 5 cc vial plus needles and syringes	not available
Premarin 1.25 mg with methyltestosterone 10 mg	$42.69 per 100	not available

◄§ *Pause and Reflect*

Gregory Goodwin Pincus is properly credited with the research that led to modern birth control pills. At about the same time he was doing this research he was also working with another group of substances that displayed strong *antihormone* properties. Doctor Pincus' unexpected early death led to a long suspension of any further study in this area. Recently, a new group of investigators has developed a marketable drug based on Doctor Pincus' original research with antihormones. Called RU 486, the drug can *obliterate* progesterone activity. It thus can serve as a birth control pill, but more importantly, it is so powerful as a progesterone inhibitor that it can regularly produce abortions in early pregnancy—up to the seventh week.

It is widely used for this purpose in other countries and is now being studied in the United States as an investigational drug under FDA guidelines. Whether or not it will ever released here for any general use is a highly controversial subject.

When testosterone is given to female canaries, it will, in about 10 days, make them sing—giving them a capability that has always been limited to male canaries.

As patents for drugs expire, consumers have been provided with more choices between brand-name (pioneer) medication and generic substitutions. As far as hormones are concerned, here are some points to consider about generics:

• Substitution laws vary from state to state. Some require substitution if the generic is cheaper, some do not. In certain states there are other laws that may affect your ability to buy generic drugs. Your pharmacist knows these regulations.

• Generics do not have to be *exact* biological equivalents to the pioneer drug. They only have to fall within 20 percent of it, one way or the other.

• Inert substances used as fillers in the generic drug may be different from those used in the pioneer drug, and may therefore cause different side effects.

• A recent study of almost 1 million prescriptions involving both pioneer and generic drugs (collected from thirty-nine states) revealed that the pharmacy *always* paid less for the generic drug; the consumer *generally* paid less for the generic than for the pioneer, but sometimes she paid *more,* and prices of generics varied widely from one pharmacy to another and a continued search was no guarantee of finding the lowest price.

It has been estimated that the routine use of hormone replacement therapy in American women would save $3.5 billion each year in medical costs. This figure was arrived at by using data developed in countries in which the regular use of HRT for the menopausal population is more widespread than it is here. The cost of regular physical examinations plus the cost of hormone therapy was subtracted from the health services provided for women with osteoporosis, arteriosclerotic heart disease and other attendant complications that develop because of hormone deficiency in the absence of hormone replacement therapy.

These data do not even attempt to address the suffering and disability that hormone-denied women suffer from their consequent medical disorders.

CHAPTER SIX

Lifestyle Advice for the Menopause

Although it is the keystone, hormone replacement therapy is only one stone supporting our menopausal and postmenopausal lives. There is a great deal more to consider, some of which we should have considered a long time ago. But, for one reason or another, we have not. Now may be our last meaningful chance to change our habits, so let's get to it. This chapter offers some lifestyle suggestions for the menopause years.

Diet

A proper diet is crucial to good health, particularly during our menopausal and postmenopausal years. Here are some observations about diet as well as material on obesity and our hyperlipid lifestyles:

• The average American diet today is far too rich in fats (40 percent or more) and sugars (23 percent) and contains twice our actual protein needs.

• Our diet is sorely deficient in fiber-rich complex carbohydrates, fruits and vegetables.

• One hundred years ago, Americans derived two-thirds of their dietary protein from low-fat starchy foods like potatoes, rice, bread, cereals, dried beans and peas, and the remaining third from meat, chicken, fish, cheese and eggs. Not so today.

• Women have been "waved off" of carbohydrates (starch) because they have been taught that carbohydrates are fattening and not nourishing. Untrue! A plain baked potato, for instance, is a nutritional bargain. For 100 calories you get protein, many nutrients and fiber. If you add butter, sour cream, cheese, bacon bits and so on, you get fat and calories and weight. And the potato, of course, gets the blame. And if you french-fry this same 100-calorie potato you have a 300-calorie megachip.

• Other great carbohydrates include rice, beans, peas and lentils. All of these are also underutilized sources of protein.

• Every plant food, however, is deficient in certain proteins and so must be combined with other plant foods in any given meal to be nutritionally complete. Generally, combining a legume (beans, pease—even peanuts) with any grain (wheat, rice, oats, etc.) makes a protein-adequate meal. Soybeans come the closest to being totally "protein-competent." Surprisingly, pizza (*good* pizza) is an excellent combination of plant and other proteins and valuable nutrients!

• Dietary fiber, which we liberally omit from our menus, comes only from plants. There are two kinds of fibers: insoluble and soluble.

Insoluble fibers, like bran, add intestinal bulk, prevent constipation and protect against colon cancer. There are three types of insoluble fibers.

There are four types of soluble fibers. These fibers slow the absorption of food, help lower cholesterol levels, decrease hunger and stabilize blood sugar levels. Thus they make excellent diet foods. They are found in whole grain breads and cereals, beans, peas, fruits and vegetables.

• Clearly, a diet inclined toward plant protein can reduce dietary fat, our most serious nutritional threat. *Fat* yields 9 calories per gram, *starch* yields only 4. Even alcohol yields only 7.

• High-fat diets are linked to increased heart disease and increased cancer of the colon, breasts and endometrium.

• There are health and weight advantages to consuming several (six) small meals a day. Fasting all night and skipping breakfast produces an inefficient, unhappy person with many metabolic problems.

• The U.S. Recommended Daily Allowances (RDAs) for women vary substantially from those of men. Women need fewer calories and less of most other nutrients, vitamins and minerals—save for iron. Menstruating women are nearly all borderline iron-deficient and require modest iron supplementation. Calcium must also be added to the daily diet once a woman reaches her middle thirties.

• A menopausal woman of average build (120 pounds) and height (5′4″) requires 1600–2400 calories daily. In the postmenopausal years (over age fifty) those needs decrease to 1400–2200 calories daily.

So where does that leave us?

The American Dietetic Society has provided women with fourteen basic suggestions (rules, they really mean) for daily dietary habits. Some of them are found in the long list below— the rest will be found on pages 81–82.

· Eat a daily variety of foods from all the major groups. Every day you should consume:

    3–4 servings from low-fat dairy group

    2 low-fat servings of meat or meat alternatives

    4 servings of vegetables and fruits

    4 servings of whole grain breads or cereals

· Total fats should make up *less* than one-third of your daily calories.

· Select fats from among a variety of sources—saturated polyunsaturated, monounsaturated—for your diet. These fats should provide only 30 percent of your daily calories—maximum—and less than 10 percent of them should be saturated fats. Read all labels.

· Limit your use of "nonfood" fats such as margarine, butter, cooking oils, salad dressings and creams.

· Choose low-fat selections from meat and dairy food groups.

· At least one-half of all your daily calories should come from carbohydrates.

· Select complex carbohydrates such as beans, peas, pasta, vegetables, nuts, seeds and rice. But avoid white bread, pancakes, waffles and the like.

• Eat a variety of fiber-rich foods: Fresh fruits with skin, vegetables and whole grains such as brown rice or oatmeal. Oat and wheat bran are also good sources of fiber.

• Increase your fiber intake gradually.

• Avoid excessive fiber intake, especially from any one source. Excess fiber can unfavorably alter the intestinal flora (the normal, healthy bacterial content of the digestive tract) and can prevent proper absorption of estrogen. So—again—more is not always better!

• Include 3–4 daily servings of calcium-rich foods in your diet: low-fat milk, yogurt, cheese, broccoli, sardines or canned salmon (with bones), greens. See page 133 for more calcium-rich foods.

• Eat iron-rich foods: lean meat, liver, prunes, pinto and kidney beans, spinach, leafy vegetables, enriched whole-grain breads and cereals and California raisins.

• Limit your intake of salt- and sodium-containing foods.

• Limit your consumption of foods already salted—ham, bacon, sausage, lunch meat, many canned foods, potato chips, crackers, etc. Read labels.

• In cooking and at the table, limit your use of salt.

• Avoid foods containing monosodium glutamate (MSG), sodium bicarbonate, sodium citrate and other sodium sources. Read labels.

• Use vitamin/mineral supplements under specific circumstances only.

• Limit alcohol to one or two drinks daily. (That can mean a lot of different things to different people. But, in your heart, you understand what this means.)

Those are the basics. You may want to consult *The American Heart Association Cookbook* and *Jane Brody's Nutrition Book* for further information.

EXCESS WEIGHT AND THE MENOPAUSE

Here are some notes on the Heavy Life.

• At any given time, over half the menopausal population claims to be on a weight-reduction diet.

• About the same number—50 percent—are truly overweight. This is so even though our generation eats less than previous generations. The problem is we move less.

• And speaking of moving less, overweight women do not necessarily eat more than their thinner counterparts, but they *move* less, even when performing the *same* tasks.

• Most popular weight-loss programs are deficient in a number of essential vitamins and minerals.

• A diet of fewer than 1200 calories is almost *never* nutritionally adequate.

• Low-calorie diets rarely produce lasting weight loss. Pounds melt away quickly at first because water is being lost. After that particular meltdown, the basal metabolic rate drops to protect the body against starvation—and that slows weight loss. Amphetamines will keep the basal metabolic rate up, but they are dangerous and addicting drugs.

• Exercise—particularly aerobic exercise—will achieve better results than starvation and drugs. Exercise raises the basal metabolic rate temporarily and, as muscle is built, raises the rate permanently. In addition, exercise burns fat.

• Studies involving identical and fraternal twins as well as adopted children reveal that there are both inherited and environmental factors in obesity development.

• As already noted, some women will gain weight on a 1200-calorie diet, some will remain the same and some will lose weight. One reason for this is the variable number of fat cells present in each individual body. The more fat cells available, the easier to gain and the harder to lose. Addressing this part of the weight-control problem requires multiple small meals, no binges and strict dietary fat restriction.

In sum, it appears that obesity is not only the first disease of modernization, it is also a very common and serious one, that is rarely due to food intake alone. Finally, most fad diets—as well as drugs—are dangerous and useless.

DIETARY GUIDELINES

If you follow these simple guidelines, you'll feel better and the menopause will pass more smoothly for you.

• Eat frequent small meals. Don't skip meals.

• Concentrate on complex carbohydrates.

• Avoid fats and empty carbohydrate calories (sugar, soda pop and alcohol, for instance).

• Eat at least 1200 nutritionally balanced calories daily. Remember, high-protein, low-carbohydrate diets lead to many problems, including irresistible carbohydrate binges.

• Always *break* your overnight *fast* with fresh whole fruits, cereals and breads. Always eat breakfast. Avoid or seriously limit caffeine in the morning and all day.

• Avoid fad diets and quick weight-loss schemes. Avoid megadoses of vitamins and minerals.

• Drink plenty of water—six to eight glasses daily. Water won't make you bloated. Sodium and sugar do that.

• *Exercise, exercise, exercise.*

The only permanent solution to weight control is a properly designed and faithfully followed lifetime eating and exercise program.

LIPIDS

Blood lipids (fats) and their elevated levels have made headline news lately. Although there are several types of blood lipids, cholesterol hogs most of the spotlight. This is because cholesterol is the one fat most likely to be elevated as a result of our dietary habits and it is the one that shingles the inside of our arteries with calcium plaques, eventually keeping our blood out and sending us to emergency rooms with heart attacks, strokes and other arterial occlusive problems.

Triglycerides, another commonly measured blood lipid, are more complex, often elevated in association with inherited disorders, gout and excess alcohol consumption and not as closely related to hardening of the arteries.

HRT helps protect women from lipid problems. Smoking makes it catastrophically worse. Dietary changes will usually restrain it.

Cholesterol is manufactured in the liver from fats the stomach gives it. Cholesterol is a very basic and desirable body building block. For instance, without cholesterol, there would be nothing for our sex glands to build sex hormones with.

Cholesterol is carried in the bloodstream by substances known as lipoproteins. There are two main types of choles-

terol carriers: high-density (HDL) and low-density (LDL) lipoproteins. HDL is considered good, or protective, while LDL
is considered bad and increases the risk of arterial disease.
Those of us with a high ratio of HDL seem to be better posi-
tioned for the long haul, and have less risk of coronary artery
disease.

Cholesterol blood levels vary within a wide range, but it
is best to have a level below 200 mg/dl (milligrams per decili-
ter). Above 240 is a worry and about 260, a red flag. The HDL
level should be 65 mg or greater.

Many foods advertised as "cholesterol-free" contain other
fats that you should avoid. One of the most common culprits
is coconut oil—a very mean saturated fat. Again, learn to read
labels.

How can you best manage your cholesterol?

• Keep your dietary fat intake *well below* 30 percent of your
total daily diet. Shoot for 20 percent.

• Make sure that both saturated and polyunsaturated fats
comprise less than 10 percent each of your daily fat intake.
Monounsaturated fats should comprise the rest. No more
than 100 mg of cholesterol should be consumed each day.
Read all labels.

• Try to consume foods that reduce cholesterol levels. Certain ocean fish contain "omega-3" fatty acids, which have the
apparent ability to increase HDL (or to decrease LDL) and
to reduce total blood cholesterol levels. Thus, concentrated
omega-3 fish oils are now being marketed heavily in this
country. The final assessment of their worth is still not in, but
you should consider adding salmon, sardines, tuna and the
like to your diet. Some green vegetables and soybean oil
contain a bit of omega-3 fatty acid as well.

• Visit your doctor. If, after proper dietary changes have been in effect for a reasonable period of time, your cholesterol levels have not returned to acceptable levels, your physician can prescribe chemical agents that may reduce blood cholesterol.

Your Personal Exercise Program

The physical activities required in daily life have vastly decreased in this century.

Machines, appliances, conveyances and conveniences have decreased our level of activity to the point where we now must manufacture, invent and prescribe things to do with our bodies in order to stay fit.

And here are some facts about exercise:

• Regular exercise, you remember, increases your basal metabolic rate by increasing your muscle mass. (Basal metabolic rate is the rate at which your body uses energy when it is at rest.) This makes it easier to keep your weight down.

• Osteoporosis can be retarded by regular exercise.

• Fitness and muscle strength increase resistance to disease (high blood pressure, diabetes, obesity, coronary artery disease), facilitate weight control and reduce tension.

• While it is true that physical activity will burn calories and help with weight control, remember that a brisk one-mile walk will expend only 100 calories, and that you must burn 3500 calories before you lose *one* pound of flesh!

Certain risks are involved in an exercise program, even a reasonable exercise program. Be aware of the following:

• Undiagnosed cardiac problems can lead to severe acute heart disorders with strenuous exercise.

• Severe—and permanent—muscle and joint injury and disease can result from the high-impact activity that is common to jogging and certain aerobic dance routines.

• Increased body core heat (hyperthermia) and excess water loss (dehydration) often follow inappropriate warm-up and cool-down programs.

Yet regular, proper exercise promotes general fitness, and involves three basic components.

1. *Aerobic endurance.* Any activity that forces the body to use more oxygen and increase the heart rate to 65 to 90 percent of maximal activity and that is engaged in for at least 20 minutes three times weekly will increase aerobic endurance. Fast walking ("wagging"), bicycling, swimming and low-impact aerobic dancing are popular ways of achieving this goal.

2. *Muscular strength.* This keeps you walking tall, protects your bony frame, and increases your metabolic rate.

3. *Joint flexibility.* This also keeps you walking tall, but in addition helps you touch your toes and scratch your back.

These three physical goals cannot be met by any one form of physical activity. So you should involve yourself in a mix of exercise activity, including walking or "wagging" or jogging, swimming, water exercises, bicycling, trampoline exercises and yoga.

These physical activities must be started slowly and followed regularly. There are many programs marketed in the United States directed toward women and their exercise needs. Many of them are dangerous and some are ineffective. The single best and safest program is on a videotape marketed (at cost) by the American College of Obstetricians and Gynecologists. Called "Balanced Fitness Workout," it can be purchased by writing:

> The American College of Obstetricians and Gynecologists
> 600 Maryland Ave. SW, Suite 300 East
> Washington, DC 20024-2258

Whatever program you settle upon should be measurably progressive and sufficiently enjoyable so that it becomes an acceptable and permanent part of your lifestyle.

No matter what degree of boredom may set into your exercise program, it will still beat a wash-tub, scrub-board, hand-wringer, clothesline and stove iron.

Habits

Most personal and intellectual habits are formed in the twenties and thirties. We are long past our twenties and even our thirties, and so all our habits—good, bad, or indifferent—are rather firmly etched and entrenched. In fact they are as much a part of us, and as difficult to erase, as the lines on our faces.

Sadly, many of our habits are destructive of our health and greatly shorten our lives and life's pleasures. We have already talked about obesity. Now, in order to continue through the menopausal successfully, we need to address some other destructive habits.

TOBACCO

Despite all you know, 35 percent of all women continue to smoke. Assuming that you don't chew tobacco, here are some points about tobacco worth remembering:

• Smoking is our nation's number one health problem. *Nothing* else comes close.

• Secondary (sidestream, passive, someone else's) smoke is probably as dangerous as your own.

• Nicotine is addictive. Like cocaine, it creates dependence and compulsive use. Nicotine use is the most widespread example of drug dependence in our country. More women now are smoking than men, so more women than men are now dying of lung cancer.

• Smoking vastly complicates hormone replacement therapy, and many gynecologists cannot recommend HRT when their patient smokes. It is well known that smokers over thirty-five who take birth control pills increase their risk of stroke and heart attacks by an *astronomical* figure. Many of us feel the same is true when women combine smoking and HRT.

• Although physicians are giving up smoking at a remarkable rate, they are *dismally* failing their patients when it comes to delivering antismoking advice. Less than half of today's doctors are counseling their patients to quit. Moreover, doctors are failing to make hospitals a smoke-free environment, which represents one of the greatest derelictions of responsibility that the medical profession can be charged with. It is like holding an AA meeting in a tavern, then treating the hangovers and charging for it!

What should you do if you smoke? You should give up smoking at once. But how can you give it up? There are two ways to quit smoking. First, make an internal resolution to quit. Nothing else is needed. Nothing else will work. Success rate? 90 percent.

If the first step doesn't work, enroll in one of the many

stop-smoking programs available in most every community. Some are free, some are expensive. About 20 percent of attendees quit smoking in the long run.

You may feel lousy for 6 to 8 months. But you will never regret it.

ALCOHOL

Former First Lady Betty Ford has stated that "alcoholism is an equal opportunity disease." And she is so right. In fact, alcoholism is now increasing at a much faster rate for women than it is for men. Many, many reasons are given for this recent phenomenon, but social and general living problems, along with lack of self-esteem, seem to head everyone's list. As in everything else, both heredity and environment play significant roles in the development of alcoholism.

The highest proportion of heavy female drinkers is found in the PeriMPX and the MPX group. Married women have the lowest overall rate and common-law wives, the highest. Most married women over fifty with alcohol problems have no children at home and do not work.

If you are burdened with unmanageable alcoholic drives, great help is available from many quarters. Alcoholics Anonymous (AA) and Women for Sobriety are two magnificent self-help groups, and many professional counselors are also available in most communities.

What about those in the menopause years who feel that they can control their relationship with alcohol? Here are some points to remember:

• If you feel *anything* about your alcohol control at all, then it is probably a problem. You can never let down your guard with alcohol. Never.

• The menopausal years are times of particular stress when alcohol dependency can slyly take over in a very unobtrusive way. Be aware of how much you drink.

• Alcohol represents empty calories that immediately join your fat system. On the way there, the alcohol tears up a few liver cells, mugs the pancreas and shakes loose some brain cells—cells that sadly are gone forever.

• One or two drinks before your evening meal are *no* problem provided that

One or two drinks before your evening meal are *no* problem.

One or two drinks means *exactly* that. One or two. (The amount of alcohol in one or two drinks should total no more than that found in two ounces of 80 proof liquor. In addition, don't mix your drink with anything but club soda or water. All other mixers contain empty, useless calories.)

None of this evening escapade was preceded by daytime trips to the bar.

You are not overweight, have no other serious health problems that may relate to alcohol consumption, and that your one or two drinks are an adjunct to a healthy, well-balanced meal.

Here is my formula for an enjoyable integration of alcohol into your lifestyle:

• You must feel that moderate alcohol intake is an integral part of the enjoyment of good living. Particularly so with good wines, which are not necessarily expensive.

• If you are in reasonably good health, you may enjoy five ounces of a light wine or blush wine with your lunch.

• Before dinner you might have one cocktail or highball. Don't mix with anything except water or club soda. Again, everything else that mixes contains empty and useless calories. At dinner, share a half carafe of an agreeable wine with an agreeable companion.

• Now that is the maximum. Nothing in the morning, no beer during the afternoon and nothing (nothing alcoholic) to get you off to bed. Anything less than the above suggestions is fine. Anything more is courting disaster.

Moderate consumption of alcohol is considered, by most medical consultants, to have positive health benefits. Alcohol is a mild tranquilizer and a reasonable mood elevator; and it can reduce blood pressure and increase organ profusion. All of which is good. Moreover, I must add, from my personal experience, there are very few lasting visceral pleasures this life has to offer that exceed that of the moderate drinking of fine wine in an appropriate setting.

Travel

As the nest empties out, more discretionary time and money may now appear on your horizon—so this may be a good time to broaden it. Today's travel opportunities are immense and this is probably the best time in your life to take advantage of them. With a few caveats.

• Be wary of sudden altitude changes. The most obvious is flying to a ski area from a much lower altitude. You are now more susceptible to altitude disorders such as mountain fever, and should spend at least one day getting used to your new environment before hitting the slopes. You will save on lift tickets and emergency room visits.

• When traveling abroad, find a good travel agent and stick to the beaten paths unless you are very adventurous, healthy, and a regular foreign traveler.

• STDs (sexually transmitted diseases) abound in many foreign countries. For example, there are 250 million new cases of gonorrhea and 25 million new cases of syphilis worldwide each year. A recent report in the *Southern Medical Journal* entitled " 'Love Boat' Hepatitis," for example, reported severe episodes of hepatitis B occurring in wealthy middle-aged women who had sexual liaisons with other passengers and crew members. So be particularly careful.

• Many other contagious and dangerous diseases lurk in foreign countries. There is a common misconception that immunization regulations set up by foreign countries are to protect the traveler. They are not. They are to protect the country. If foreign governments were interested in *your* health, they would publish their national disease statistics in their travel brochures. If you want the real scoop about the disease risks in foreign lands, contact the United States Public Health Service.

• Hopefully your food will have been harvested long *after* your wine but, just in case, be wary of wayside inns.

• If you plan to live in another country for an extended period of time you should ask the United States Public Health Service for its list of vaccines appropriate for that country.

• The International Association for Assistance to Travelers, 350 Fifth Avenue, New York, NY 10001, will, for a fee, provide you with a list of English-speaking physicians almost anywhere abroad.

• Remember how to manage jet lag: much water, little alcohol and light eating on board and rest on arrival. Better to travel by ship.

• Take an extra, separate supply of your medications. When possible, leave all of them in their original bottles, clearly labeled with your name and the contents as written by your pharmacist. Some foreign customs agents take a dim view of unlabeled medications mixed together like jelly beans. Pack your original medications in your carry-on luggage and your backup supplies elsewhere.

All in all, have a nice trip.

Wellness and Fulfillment

This menopause book would not serve you properly without discussing the concept of total body wellness. The bedrock of good health is the integration of a well-managed body with a well-ordered spirit (psyche, soul—whatever you wish to call it). And, in the order of things, the spirit compartment is dominant. A strong and directed spiritual will to live and to control the flow and exuberance of bodily activity is the key to total wellness.

How is this spiritual goal achieved? Well, purposeful living requires us all to examine and consider the likely existence of a greater force in our lives and in the universal order than we can readily explain, a force that constantly provides us with a dependable and abiding haven (something we cannot provide for each other or that cannot be provided for us by creature comforts or visceral pleasures). Call this a spiritual force or whatever you will. Approach it by any rational religious or philosophical bridge you choose.

If you accept it you are well on your way to a dominant spiritual life, without which there cannot be total wellness and with which all things are possible.

This is valuable advice for the menopausal years and those that follow. Many of you already understand these things.

❧ *Pause and Reflect*

Excess caffeine intake (caffeinism) produces a type of anxiety very common in women. Too often the cause goes unrecognized and improper treatment (tranquilizers, for instance) is prescribed. Gradual withdrawal from the culprit (coffee, tea, soft drinks and chocolate) is the proper treatment and essential to good health.

Caffeine is also linked directly to other health problems—some of them deadly. A recent study in the *New England Journal of Medicine* demonstrates a two- to threefold increase in heart attacks among adults drinking five or more cups of coffee daily.

Always read labels! The United States government requires that all enriched or fortified foods and all foods that make nutritional claims be labeled with nutritional information. Two types of information may be listed. Get out a milk carton and follow along.

• First, the "Nutrition Information per Serving" is listed. This shows the calories per serving as well as the protein, carbohydrates and fats present. Although not required, some producers will list the amount of cholesterol and the various types of fats present.

• Second, the percentages of Recommended Daily Allowances (US RDAs) are also listed. Some of these (iron, for instance) must be listed; others are up to the manufacturer.

Not all foods are labeled. Fresh fruits and vegetables, fresh meats, fishes and poultry clearly cannot be labeled. Their values are easily obtained from any book listing food values.

————————

The average American gets over 100 times the amount of daily sodium required.

————————

Fat men are more likely to be sick than fat women. Moreover, women with male-like obesity (upper body fat) are more likely to be sick than women with lower-body obesity.

————————

Women's fat deposits are harder to mobilize and reduce than are men's. This is because men have a higher concentration of a fat-mobilizing hormone.

————————

The amount of time that a child between six and eleven years of age spends before a television set is the most powerful predictor of his or her adolescent obesity.

————————

Supplemental vitamins and minerals often interact with other nutrients, particularly in the megadose range. For instance, large doses of calcium taken throughout the day may interfere with iron absorption.

The effect of alcohol upon sexual arousal and pleasure for women has been the subject of jokes, locker-room discussions and sophomoric conjecture for ages. But a closely controlled study shows that women who thought they had consumed alcohol felt more aroused, whether they had been given alcohol or not. Conversely, women who actually consumed alcohol had less and less arousal as they increased their consumption of liquor.

CHAPTER SEVEN

The Menopause and the Bedroom

Sleep

A good night's sleep during the menopause, as at all other times of your life, is very important. One of the first good sleep principles is to be very careful what gets between the sheets with you at night. You must learn to empty your mind of the frustrations, fears, and angers that the day has heaped upon you. Bring them in with you and they'll irritate you all night and still be there in the morning. Believe me, you *can* learn to put them out with the cat.

Certain things work against your chances of a good sleep at menopause time. By far the most common is, of course, night sweats. Night sweats are almost totally preventable by adequate hormone replacement therapy.

Here are some more sleep helpers:

  • Use your bedroom for sleeping and loving only. Put your TV set elsewhere. No reading, writing, knitting or TV watching in bed.

• Go to bed when you are sleepy but try to get up at about the same time each morning. Even if you have slept poorly, try not to nap during the day.

• As I said, leave the thoughts, torments, and events of the day behind, and fantasize. That can mean anything from counting sheep to counting the hairs on Casanova's chest. Boring fantasies (like the sheep) seem to work better for some individuals than do the exciting ones. Use any fantasy that gets you involved and that works for you.

• Avoid exercise (except sex), caffeine, and alcohol after you finish your evening meal. Alcohol may relax you into falling asleep, but the sleep is usually not deep or lasting.

• Avoid dependency on sleeping preparations of any kind.

• "White noise" sometimes helps a poor sleeper drop off pleasantly. Such things as ceiling fans, tapes of rainstorms and safe-harbor and seashore sounds often have this effect. They also serve to block out unwanted background noise—like someone else's TV, cat, dog, or snoring.

• Don't eat just before retiring or retire just after eating.

• If all else fails, visit a sleep clinic. Little Rock, which is a small city, has at least three sleep clinics, so these clinics are not uncommon. Most audiovisual stores rent sleep-training tapes, or can get them for you.

Sex and Loving

A great revolution has occurred in our sexual lives and attitudes since the days when a British mother's only advice for her betrothed daughter was "Close your eyes and think of England." The revolution has brought many changes—some bad, most good—in our sexual activities and customs. One of the best changes involves women's freedom to develop and experience their own uninhibited and unfettered sexual expression and pleasure. Now, as the menopausal and postmenopausal ranks swell, questions about continued sexuality become increasingly common.

Menopausal women can expect several changes that normally take place as time goes by. For example, a woman's sex drive often rises somewhat at MPX as ovarian estrogen levels drop while androgen (a male-like hormone) levels persist. This is not always the case and certainly not true if the menopause has been surgically induced and the ovaries are absent. Sexual desire continues in women (but at decreasing levels as the years go by), and is not at all unusual in women in their seventies and eighties.

Testosterone is available for those women who suffer from a significant loss of sexual drive during and after a natural or surgical menopause. Proper dose levels of this male hormone—in combination with estrogen—will generally prevent excess hair growth and other masculinizing effects. Regular medical monitoring and dose adjustment is necessary.

Excitement and arousal, which are usually marked by vaginal lubrication and swelling, also change. Sexual arousal now often requires more foreplay and local stimulation; indeed, without HRT, natural lubrication may not be possible. In addition, if HRT is absent, vaginal skin atrophy occurs and leads to painful intercourse along with many other local discomforts. You've read about this already.

Orgasm continues but "time-to-orgasm" may be lengthened without HRT. Menopausal and PMPX women may continue to experience multiple orgasms as before.

Yet there are several other factors in your new sexual equation. First, what about him? If he is your partner of long standing and about your age, his sex drive started declining several years ago and will diminish more rapidly than yours. In addition, although about 80 percent of seventy- to eighty-year-old men claim sexual activity, arousal takes much longer, and usually involves some form of direct stimulation of the penis along with great care to achieve and maintain erection. These changes, mind you, are gradual in onset. Finally, the latent time between successful orgasms increases so that by age sixty, male orgasm cannot be repeated for about 2 days. This is sharply different from the female's experience. While testosterone medication will increase men's drive somewhat, it does not increase their erectile or orgasmic ability.

It is clear that many diseases can and will hasten the usual aging changes in sexual activity of both men and women. Diabetes, high blood pressure, obesity, arthritis and heart disease are common medical obstructions to sexual pleasure. Men who have suffered one heart attack often fear that sexual activity may induce another one. That understandable fear may decrease the level of performance, even though studies indicate sexual exertion to orgasm is the exercise-equivalent of walking up one flight of stairs. It is worth noting, though, that 70 percent of the sex-related heart attack deaths occur during an *extramarital* event!

Many of the medications necessary to maintain reasonable health at mid-life act as sexual depressants. These include drugs for anxiety and depression, heart disease, high blood pressure and fluid retention. Sedatives and many others also have this effect. The only valuable medications for women, sexually speaking, are the sex hormones—HRT.

Alcohol abuse is a serious and common cause of sexual dysfunction for both sexes.

The last, and perhaps most important, factor in your new sexual equation is the quality of your partnership. This is really the key to a rich—or barren—sexual life. All of the factors noted above, taken together, depend upon the depth and stability of the union along with an understanding of the changes that accompany aging. An unstable relationship filled with pent-up angers and frustrations will surely fly apart at this time. A healthy, mature, growing relationship will be able to explore more erotic and sensual sexual depths than ever before.

How Best to Approach Sexuality in the Menopause and Beyond

Remember what you just read, particularly two things: first, your same-aged mate will likely be undergoing a decline in sexual drive more rapidly than you. Second, this is particularly true if you are being supported by HRT and he is not. At the present time, HRT (testosterone, in this case) is not generally recommended for men.

If both partners understand the age-related changes that normally take place at mid-life, they will be more likely to prevent serious sexual and marital problems down the line. Thus, as an example, if you both understand that it now takes direct stimulation of his genitals (orally, mechanically, thermally, digitally, or whatever it takes) in order to produce an erection, then no one's feelings are hurt. *You* don't feel you have lost your appeal and *he* doesn't feel that sex, as he knew it, is over.

On the above basis, minor sexual problems can generally be worked out at home in bed. Major sexual problems that occur at this time are generally a result of serious disorders in your relationship and require professional sex and marriage counseling.

Vaginal penetration is neither the beginning nor the end of sexual lovemaking. It sometimes cannot be accomplished—

at any age. Shared intimacy, sensual pleasure, holding and caressing are often equally meaningful and enjoyable.

Sex should not be performance-oriented, but rather pleasure-oriented. For both of you. Together you should seek an erotic arousal environment, comfortable to both, with no demands and only the exploration of new pleasures.

Special Situations

Some special situations may affect the ways in which you express your sexuality. For instance:

• May-December relationships require special attention. If your loved one is much older than you, it is necessary that you make generous allowances for his sexual limitations which, as you are aware, are real and progressive.

• If your spouse becomes permanently impotent because of medical or other reasons, and if it is the wish of both partners, penile implants are now a reasonable solution. However, without any help, many older men remain sexually active and erectile well into their eighties.

• Now, then, the reverse. A much younger husband, biologically, should be the ideal sexual companion for a mid-life woman. That is probably the case, although I do not have the statistics to prove it. What *is* proven, though, is that the nonsexual complications of this kind of relationship are difficult to maintain.

• Surgical or radiation treatment for cancer of the breasts or of the uterus can have profound effects upon future sexual activity. As you already know, hormone replacement cannot be given for at least five years after arrested cancer of the breast or the uterus. Thus the vagina becomes dry and painful and sex drive is diminished. Some physicians will give oral testosterone or vaginal estrogen creams, but most fear the consequences in the patient—or in court.

Removal of a breast or other massive disfigurement of the sexual organs has a very understandable emotional impact. Fortunately, in almost every community, there are now support groups made up of women who have sustained ostomies and mastectomies and destructive vulvovaginal surgery, and who very successfully counsel others who join their support group. In most instances, adequate professional counseling and the judicious use of hormones will alleviate the most distressing circumstances. Partners can be instructed in a variety of loving techniques as time heals the psyche.

Loners

Some women live alone by choice, but an increasing number find themselves alone as a result of being widowed, divorced or separated. In any case, sexuality and normal sexual drives remain a fact of life that must be dealt with. Women who live alone by choice have already met that problem one way or another. The newly divorced or widowed woman at mid-life has but few choices to resolve her new problem.

Masturbation is a safe, harmless way to release sexual energy and pressure. Any nonirritating lubricant and a vibrator are all that is needed. Masturbation is not immoral, unnatural or dangerous.

There is a pack of predators skulking in the wings waiting to help newly divorced or widowed women to continue their sexual life. Members of this happy little band of do-gooders not only carry with them the desire to help you obtain continued sexual relief, but may also carry with them every known sexually transmitted disease. Which is about the only thing you will get out of the relationship. Watch out for these men.

Forming meaningful new relationships has its own problems too. Multiple relationships are dangerous, if for no other reason than health. Remember, a condom covers only the penis. The mouth and hands and everything else lie bare and can carry disease.

Even forming a relationship that you wish to be continuing and monogamous can be dangerous insofar as sexually transmitted diseases are concerned. Any male interested in you has probably been interested in and active with other women. It is a difficult challenge to face. And I don't have the answer. Today, there probably is no answer.

Lesbians

Relationships between lesbian women are much more stable than those of male homosexuals. Since sexual aging and drive generally proceeds at the same rate in a lesbian relationship, there is much less likelihood of sexual disharmony than in a heterosexual relationship. Another interesting point: Lesbian women complain much less of menopausal symptoms than do their heterosexual counterparts.

Sexually Transmitted Diseases at Mid-Life

In today's sexual climate, concerns about STDs (sexually transmitted diseases) during and after the menopause years are understandable, particularly when we read that 10 percent of all female AIDS victims are over fifty!

Monogamous couples have no need to fear AIDS—unless one of them injects IV drugs or does work that brings her (or him) into contact with blood or other body fluids from AIDS patients. People working in these environments are acutely aware of the hazards and protective responsibilities. AIDS contracted by blood transfusion is now extremely rare.

Nondrug-abusing monogamous couples need have no fear of contacting any sexually transmitted diseases unless one of the partners is an asymptomatic carrier of an STD from a previous relationship. Of the STDs, herpes and condylomata (genital warts)—both viruses—are the two most commonly transmitted at present. In this regard, the incidence of genital herpes is rising dramatically in MPX women. Whether or not this represents changing sexual patterns in this age group of women is not now known. But it is a fact. Fortunately, most MPX women appear to have built up an immunity to condylomata over the years and this infection is not very often seen in this age group.

Of the bacterial STDs, chlamydia, gonorrhea and syphilis are all increasing in the MPX population, but at a slower rate than the virus infections. And they are generally easier to treat. The symptoms, signs and treatment of these STDs are far beyond the scope of this book. But any unusual discharges, ulcers, sores, growths, warts, redness or swellings in the vaginal and rectal areas need prompt medical attention.

Most times, when you ask a new partner about his sexual disease history, you will hear what he wants you to hear. Nothing else. And remember, safe sex is not just having your partner wear a condom, since it covers only his penis, which is but a tiny part of his sexual equipment. Safe sex is a longstanding monogamous relationship.

Birth Control

Although research has indicated that couples become infertile when the woman reaches about forty years of age, don't depend upon it. I have delivered many babies for women well into their forties.

What is true is that fertility in the forties is vastly diminished by reduced sexual activity, declining male sperm counts and irregular and infrequent ovulation.

Even though the likelihood of pregnancy is reduced, very few women at menopause have active reproductive goals, so concerns about birth control are very real.

Sterilization has become the birth control method of choice for both men and women during the past twenty years as techniques have become simpler and safer. Today about 30 percent of women and 15 percent of men choose surgical sterilization as their method of birth control. And it rarely fails.

Modern low-dosage birth control pills are, for nonsmoking, otherwise healthy women, a safe, reliable method of menopausal birth control. Not only that, the newer birth control pills that contain very low doses of estrogen or estrogen-like substances plus progesterone offer proven protection against endometrial cancer, ovarian tumors, ectopic pregnancies, pelvic infections and iron-deficiency anemia. And just as with our regular HRT programs, these pills do not increase the risk of breast cancer; in fact, they probably decrease it. Thus, for nonsmoking women, the birth control pill not only acts as an excellent contraceptive but as a hormone replacement therapy as well, all the while producing health dividends. All such programs must be closely monitored with regular blood pressure and blood lipid tests.

The intrauterine contraceptive device (IUD) is currently being remarketed in the United States after a brief marketing withdrawal because one type of IUD was harmful. IUDs are a good MPX contraceptive for three reasons: they are very effective in the MPX age group; concerns about long-term fertility effects are nonexistent; and as menopausal women are less likely to have multiple sexual partners, there is less risk of pelvic infections with the IUD.

In view of the generally decreased fertility at MPX, condoms and diaphragms offer excellent contraceptive protection. Other barriers are less effective.

WHEN TO QUIT?

When should you stop using birth control? The answer must come from your own gynecologist.

Generally speaking, oral contraceptives—as well as HRT—will make women continue to have regular cycles long after they are no longer fertile. Stop the hormones and the periods will stop. But, of course, you don't want to stop the hormones. Sooner or later, however, you will want to switch from OCs to regular HRT. HRT is a generally adequate, though not proven, contraceptive for women from the mid-forties on.

IUDs may safely be removed and barrier contraceptives safely pitched after one year of amenorrhea (no periods). Most are generally discontinued before that time.

◄§ *Pause and Reflect*

Two potential birth control ideas in the works may be of interest to you: First, an "electrical fence" device that is designed to zap sperm as they attempt to swim by. This is a mechanical device, implanted into the cervix on a long-term basis, which carries a very minor electrical current (batteries included).

What do you think satin sheets—or an electric blanket—will do to that charged encounter? Second, scientists are working on a nasal spray that men can use daily to suppress sperm production. Unfortunately, it also suppresses testosterone production, so subcutaneous pellets of that vital male hormone must be used in conjunction with the nose spray to keep men at the ready.

The Hutterites are a very religious and moral sect that migrated into this country and Canada in the last century. They do not believe in birth control, and because they marry within their own ranks, they offer scientists an excellent opportunity to study declining fertility under natural circumstances and in a very healthy population. Studies indicate a marked and steady decrease in fertility after thirty in the Hutterites. In addition, the mean age of last live birth in this type of population preceded the menopause by about 10 years.

Insofar as AIDS is concerned, the surest sexual way of transmitting it is by anal intercourse. This is not an uncommon sexual practice in our society; 238 of 723 women interviewed in 1987 about their sexual practices were active anal-intercourse participants. To protect yourself against AIDS you should avoid anal sex.

In the discussion on sexuality you learned that women's sex drive lasts well into the seventies and beyond. In one study, 20 percent of women interviewed at age seventy-five expressed continuing sexual interest. Most women with continuing sexual interest at this time of life weigh significantly more than the noninterested. It is believed that their extra fat stores more estrogen, which, in turn, stimulates sexual arousal.

Sleeping and sleep disorders are very much more complicated than my short discussion would indicate. At least one-third of all Americans have some sort of sleeping problem. Over 40 million prescriptions are written each year for sleeping pills. Believe it or not, that represents a great reduction from the number written in a year a decade ago.

Modern sleeping pills, which are said to have a short half-life in the body, are now believed to have prolonged and sustained effects. The most important appears to be memory loss—something that often happens during the menopausal years and that doesn't need to be supplemented by drugs.

For more sleep information read *The American Medical Association Guide to Better Sleep* by Lynne Lambert (Random House, 1984).

CHAPTER EIGHT

The Postmenopause

This state fills the rest of your life. It includes the immediate postmenopausal years and leads to your "Master Citizen" life—sometimes called the Third Life, the Golden Years, Senior Citizenship and more. In reality you will become a Master Citizen with all its rights and privileges—which mainly consist of back-handing the government, getting off committees, doing your own thing while enjoying your quirks, straightening out your doctor and being a great deal wiser than the next 100 people you meet.

You will be postmenopausal until you join the final exodus. That may take another forty years. You had better pay attention to the following information, since it will probably involve one-third to one-half of your life.

First of all, you can rejoice in the fact that modern medical technology has rendered these years productive, healthy and fulfilling. It is true that time exacts its toll and the aging process continues until it masters us all, but the following advice will make your postmenopausal years exhilarating, prolonged and trouble-free.

What should you do about your HRT program? First, recall the basic four reasons for instituting HRT: to protect and preserve your sexuality, to arrest or delay osteoporosis, to protect your cardiovascular system and to control flushes, sweats, insomnia and emotional storms.

Flushes, sweats and the like generally diminish, and osteoporosis slows in most women after a few years. But osteoporosis does not stop. Neither does arteriosclerosis. And sexuality continues to decline. Again, HRT gently slows all these aging processes with benefits that vastly outweigh the risks. So, whenever possible, HRT, in some form, should be continued.

HRT Programs for the Postmenopause

The duration of progesterone administration in each cycle is generally increased as the years go by for three reasons: first, if the uterus is still in place, the added progesterone (given in the form of a progestin) tends to make menstruation disappear in time. A welcome relief. Second, progesterone, it now appears, tends to build new bone. Estrogen only delays loss of old bone. And finally, there is increasing—but not absolute—evidence that progesterone helps protect breast tissue against cancer.

The limited negative effect that small doses of progestins have on lipid metabolism (see page 82) is now thought to be balanced by the beneficial effect of estrogen. So the increase in progesterone apparently poses no significant added risk—at the most, a trade-off.

Testosterone is added to the HRT program because it enhances sexuality. The dose must be carefully controlled to prevent unwanted masculinizing effects (excessive hair growth, voice changes, clitoral enlargement, etc.) but this can and is being done. Usually the testosterone is given by mouth, but administration via pellets implanted under the skin is now available. About 20 percent of all PMPX patients seem to benefit from this added therapy. That number may increase significantly as more women recognize the value and availability of testosterone therapy and open up about their sexual needs.

The ovaries produce testosterone and testosterone-like hormones throughout their active life. After the menopause some ovaries continue producing small amounts of these hormones, which continue to enhance sex drive. Surgical removal of the ovaries obliterates the primary mechanism for the production of male-like hormones in a woman's body (although a certain amount of these hormones continues to be manufactured in the adrenal glands). Thus, testosterone is often added to regular HRT for women who have surgically lost their ovaries.

Estrogen is more likely to be given parenterally (not by mouth) in the PMPX as we gain more confidence in these techniques. This method, then, would include shots, subcutaneous (under the skin) pellets and skin patches. Skin patches of estrogen are now very common and have virtually no side effects other than skin irritation in some individuals. Estrogen given transdermally (across the skin) in this manner is less likely to cause high blood pressure than is estrogen given by the oral route. On the other hand, we cannot say that it prevents osteoporosis because it will take years to prove that point to everyone's satisfaction. It is worth noting, however, that when you obtain a blood level of estradiol from some a woman, you cannot tell whether that estradiol came from her ovary, a pill, a shot, a skin patch, a vaginal suppository, or a pellet. Neither can the body. Neither can the bone.

In many parts of the world, and in a few places in the United States, a pellet or pellets of estradiol, implanted under the skin, are being used as the regular mode of HRT. Oral progestins may be used concurrently since there are, as yet, no available progestin pellets. At any rate, the pellet is implanted under the skin (preceded by a local anesthetic), usually just above the pubic hairline. The pellet provides smooth and adequate levels of estradiol for up to 6 months. A new one is then put in place. As you already know, a testosterone pellet can be inserted at the same time.

There are still some problems to be worked out with this HRT program, but it is coming on strong and may be the wave of the immediate future.

As the postmenopausal years march along, HRT is reduced to the least effective level of the involved hormones. But no one yet knows when, if ever, it should be discontinued. Many gynecologists are continuing HRT for women into their seventies and eighties. Factors to be considered are the need and the risks.

The threat of progressive arteriosclerosis, the continuing threat of osteoporosis in susceptible women, the woman's desire to maintain an active sexual life, and other continued needs for hormone support must be considered when deciding whether or not to continue HRT. In addition, the risks must be considered. The possibility of cancer of the uterus or the breasts, along with the possibility of phlebitis, high blood pressure, unknown distant effects and absence of needs, all must be considered when deciding upon HRT fold-up time. As in everything else, it should be a mutual decision between physician and patient.

Lifestyle Advice for the Postmenopause

As in the menopause, certain guidelines must be followed for better health in the postmenopause.

EXERCISE

Regardless of how good you feel and how hard you work at your health goals, aging is relentless. Thus, your heart output drops by 8 percent every ten years, your lung capacity decreases, your blood pressure tends to rise and your arteries get harder. Further, muscles weaken and joints stiffen, decreasing your mobility and power. Your bone mass decreases, even on HRT.

If you stay on your HRT program, all these aging problems are delayed—but you inevitably have to adjust to them. One way to adjust is through exercise. The basic philosophy of your postmenopausal physical exercise program is outlined in Chapter 6. The three main activity groups—aerobics, flexing and muscle strengthening—should all be continued, unless some physical problem intervenes and forces a shutdown. Continue your exercising at least three times weekly. You can do it.

Remember, walking, swimming, and bicycling remain excellent aerobic exercises for you. Yoga may be a new way for you to increase flexibility and relaxation.

Remember the enemy: inertia, the tendency of a body to remain at rest. Keep moving!

DIET

The menopausal diet outlined in Chapter 6 needs little alteration as you march along. There are a few changes as you age, however.

Your caloric intake must be gradually reduced since your needs will constantly decline. Most physicians agree that, depending upon your body frame and your activity level, you should aim for 1400–2200 calories daily. About 25 percent of this should be fat—proper fat.

Avoid highly seasoned foods. They become harder and harder to digest, so that after a four-alarm chili meal you may feel like you have just swallowed the world.

Decrease your intake of smoked foods and salty foods. Smoked foods increase your risk of cancer and salty foods increase your risk of high blood pressure.

Be sure you get your daily allotment of calcium and daily vitamins. Extra iron will not be so important if you are no longer menstruating and have no other blood loss disorder.

Include fiber in your meal. Reread the section about fiber foods and their different values in Chapter 6. Whole fresh fruits and vegetables are important and so is bran. And now there is evidence that even Metamucil will help lower your cholesterol level as well as supply you with safe, virtually calorie-free bulk.

TOBACCO

If you continue to smoke, keep trying to break the habit. Every drag you avoid lengthens your life and the quality of it. Now, sad to say, is when the lifelong tobacco habit begins to round up its victims. Thus heart disease, strokes, emphysema and cancer—not only of the lungs but of many other body sites—begin their march across our lives. Stop smoking.

ALCOHOL

The abuse of alcohol is almost as deadly as the use of nicotine and tends to increase in women, for multiple reasons, in the postmenopausal years. Excellent help is available from AA and other support sources in almost every community. Meanwhile, a bottle of beer, a glass or two of wine or a drink of whiskey can be stimulating and relaxing—even healthful—to any of you who like alcohol and have no contraindicating health problems. Just don't offend or tempt nature or make a meal of alcohol.

SLEEP

Regardless of what you hear, you will always need the amount of sleep your body has been accustomed to. You may begin to awaken earlier for a number of reasons, but that simply means you will have to retire earlier. If possible, however, it is better to maintain your regular sleep patterns, retiring and rising as usual. In reality, as time goes by, sleeping becomes less of a problem.

MEDICINE

Recent studies involving some 25,000 United States physicians (including me) strongly indicate that an aspirin tablet taken every other day reduces the risk of myocardial infarction (heart attack) by almost 50 percent! For five years, half of the participating doctors took a placebo and half took an aspirin every other day, none of us knowing what we were getting. The placebo group (which included me) had twice as many heart attacks. I'm now on aspirin.

At any rate, aspirin works this particular magic by decreasing the rate at which blood usually clots, thus allowing it to flow more freely through hardened constricted arteries. Since this factor would also tend to prevent clot formation in phlebitis and other vein disturbances, aspirin may be a very valuable agent in these problems as well. Thus, for a number of reasons, an aspirin every other day could join our postmenopausal medicine chest. Don't start on your own, though. Check with your doctor. And remember: *More is not better.*

Fulfillment

The firm base of friends and family that you have built will support you in all your encounters—good and bad—as your postmenopausal years unfold. There will be adversity through death, separation, divorce, illness, finances and loneliness. These temporal things can strike us at any time in our lives, but they multiply as we age. A lot of pleasurable and memorable things will also happen to us and so the good and the bad must be integrated and handled. So here is your plan:

. Keep a circle of friends and keep interacting with them positively. A social network is a net that will catch you in a crisis.

Define meaningful goals for the future. Don't knit or do social, civic or community chores because you have nothing else to do. Do it because it is fulfilling for you—or do something else that is. There are thousands of things you can do.

When grief over a loss strikes you, let the natural grieving process unfold and run its course. Share your feelings with the various members of your network as they will share theirs with you. It helps. Speaking of help, it may be necessary, if grieving overwhelms you, to seek professional counseling. Don't delay accepting such help. There is no stigma attached to it.

Continue to interact with your gynecologist/physician on a regular basis—at least once a year, preferably twice a year. Why?

- Your HRT needs to be constantly updated.

- Mammogram and bone density studies need monitoring.

- Regular Pap smears are important. Even with your uterus gone, you need a Pap smear every few years. With your uterus still in you need one every year, regardless of what you hear.

• A general physical examination with appropriate lab work will help you avoid degenerative changes, high blood pressure, heart disorders, serious gynecological disease, and so on.

• Your doctor is—or should be—a part of your network as well as a counselor.

• This is a time when serious disorders of your pelvic organs are on the increase. Close and regular observation can only help in early detection and successful management.

Let's look at three malignancies of the pelvic organs that are more likely to appear in the postmenopausal years.

Cancer of the vulva appears as skin changes follow aging and estrogen deprivation. Close observation and monitoring by modern colposcopic techniques can lead to treatment that can, in many cases, reverse, halt or correct such disorders before radical surgery must be undertaken to remove an actual cancer of the vulva.

Cancer of the endometrium is rarely seen before the menopause and usually many years afterwards. Again, close observation and biopsies at the slightest sign of postmenopausal bleeding help establish an early diagnosis. When endometrial cancer is diagnosed early, the arrest rates approach 95 percent. Moreover, many physicians are providing postmenopausal women with a provocative or challenge progesterone test every 6 to 12 months after the menses have ceased. In this test, a measured amount of progesterone (in the form of a progestin) is given over a week's time. In order for progesterone given as progestins to produce menstrual bleeding, there must be some activity in the uterine endometrial lining.

Postmenopausally, if no estrogen is being administered, there should be absolutely no such endometrial activity at all. Thus, if the administration of a progestin does bring on any type of menstrual bleeding within a month after its administration, it must be assumed that some abnormal activity is present in the endometrium and that activity must be clearly identified by biopsy or by a D&C (dilatation and curettage) operation. As this challenge procedure becomes more widespread, it may allow the detection of early dangerous endometrial changes before they become invasive cancers. Remember that this same progesterone challenge test is also used to help determine the degree of ovarian failure in younger women. This has been described in Chapter 2.

Cancer of the ovaries is among the most feared of all female pelvic cancers, mainly because it is very hard to detect except in its advanced stages. Regular pelvic examinations, coupled with ultrasound inspection of the ovaries, offer us the greatest hope of conquering this particular cancer. Other, better, techniques are on the way, but this is the best we have to offer today.

All in all, then, you need to put your doctor into your postmenopausal network program, interaction group, or involvement program. Spend some quality time with her.

◄§ Pause and Reflect

Postmenopausal women often experience a fractured wrist long before they begin to lose bone density in any significant amount. This accident appears to be a result of women putting out their hands to break a fall. Thus, evidence now points to the fact that, because of their increased postural sway, more menopausal women fall inadvertently, and that this particular fracture results from that fall, not from increased bone fragility.

————————

Recent evidence indicates that women on postmenopausal HRT have better long-term memories and greater concentration powers than their nonHRT sisters.

CHAPTER NINE

Osteoporosis

All of a sudden, it seems, osteoporosis has become an overwhelming issue in your health management. But, in actuality, that is not so. The subject, along with the disorder itself, has been approaching us gradually, gathering momentum like the ever-rolling surf, until it now threatens to break upon us with force sufficient to crumble and wash away a vast number of our Master Citizens. It has become a very "in" subject to discuss. It has also become a very compelling medical problem, a problem related to the immense increase of women's lifespan.

Remember, osteoporosis is a reduction in the quantity of bony material in the body. It causes structural weakness and increased fragility of the bones—mainly by the loss of bone calcium—and predisposes the bearer to certain fractures. Although there are several types of osteoporosis, with different causes, this section is concerned only with osteoporosis that strikes postmenopausal women and is related to bone calcium loss initiated by the absence of estrogen.

To give you just a glimpse into the magnitude of the osteoporosis cataclysm, here are some vital statistics:

• The disorder will eventually affect *every other* postmenopausal woman.

• One in three postmenopausal women will have a fracture sooner or later.

• There are in the United States 250,000 hip fractures in postmenopausal women each year. This will increase (unless we change our ways) to 500,000 by the end of this century.

• Of these women with hip fractures, 17% will die within 3 months, 40% within 6 months. Among survivors, 75% will lose their independence and 25% will require skilled nursing care.

• Eight out of every hundred of women now thirty-five years old can expect to end up with a hip fracture sooner or later. Usually later. At least one-third of all women over ninety have sustained a hip fracture.

• Osteoporosis costs us about $10 billion now and will cost us over $30 billion by the year 2000 unless we change our ways.

• Twenty-five percent of all women over sixty have spinal compression fractures. This will rise to 50 percent before they are ninety.

The Bare Bone Facts

Physicians used to take great pride in exhibiting a full skeleton hanging prominently in their consultation rooms. The purpose of the skeleton was not very clear, but it did clearly reveal that the human frame was, indeed, made up of several hundred fairly uniform-looking bones that seemed very hard and unalterable. Thus we all came away with the impression that the skeleton, made up of bones, was a fixed and permanent affair—much like the steel girders of a bridge.

Regardless of what we saw, however, our bony frame is not the least bit fixed and unalterable. It is a living and dynamic support system that is in constant change and that responds to many hundreds of variable stimulations, both good and bad, some building, some destroying. The commonest destroyer is osteoporosis, and it is second only to arthritis as the leading cause of disability amongst Master Citizens.

Here, then, is what you need to know about bone. Bone begins to form in embryos at about 12 weeks and continues to grow and develop for about twenty years. By that time our frame is generally complete and only the bone density may be altered.

There are two basic kinds of bone: cortical and trabecular. *Cortical* bone is the smooth exterior solid shaft that is visible on the surface of all bones. *Trabecular* bone is that found within the cortical sheath and is, in appearance, honeycombed. This very important bone functions like the small girders you see holding massive iron beams in place, keeping them from buckling. It is important to remember these two types of bone since they disappear at different times after the menopause.

Bone, under normal circumstances, is constantly being removed (by cells called osteoclasts) and constantly being rebuilt (by osteoblasts). This constant changing is called *remodeling*. Living bone is never at metabolic rest so it is constantly remodeling at an annual rate ranging from 50 percent in a 2-year-old to 5 percent in an adult.

Normal and stable bone remodeling is controlled by many factors. Bone growth is stimulated by weight-bearing activity, sex hormones, pituitary growth hormones and normal thyroid activity. Bone loss is increased by physical inactivity, by excess adrenal hormones (corticosteroids) or thyroid hormones and by parathyroid activity, which is involved in calcium regulation, as well as by the absence of sex hormones, particularly estrogen.

Bone mass peaks between thirty and forty; proper diet and exercise will ensure that you have a maximum, stable, strong frame to carry you into the PMPX years.

As indicated above, women begin to experience bone loss in their thirties—even before menopausal symptoms develop. During the five to ten years that follow the menopause, a dramatic acceleration of bone loss begins—first the trabecular bone (which supports the vertebrae), and then, at a later date, the cortical bone. Thus, collapsed vertebrae, with the attendant pain and height loss are usually the first clinical sign of osteoporosis.

·One of the functions of bone is to store calcium for use when other bodily processes require it. These storage functions are regulated by certain cells of the thyroid glands, which secrete extra calcitonin when bone stores are being drained.

Let's look at an average person's daily calcium metabolism, remembering that this mineral needs to be kept in strict internal balance not only for bone strength but for all normal body functions.

Calcium comes into the body from dietary and supplementary sources. It leaves the body through the intestines and the kidneys. Obviously, for balance, the intake must equal the outgo. Each day the kidneys filter 8,000 mg of calcium and loose 200 mg in the process. The intestines also lose another 300 mg of calcium each day. Thus, 500 mg of pure calcium must be absorbed from food and supplements each day to maintain balance.

Now then, to absorb 500 mg of pure calcium daily, it would be necessary to consume over 1,000 mg of various calcium salts; but the average American diet provides only 650 mg. Thus, supplementation is almost always necessary—to the tune of at least 350 mg of pure calcium each day. Of the common supplementary calcium salts, calcium carbonate is 40 percent calcium, calcium lactate is 13 percent, calcium gluconate is 9 percent and calcium citrate is 30 percent calcium. Thus, if you use calcium carbonate (Tums, for instance) as your supplement, you would need to take at least 800 mg each day.

As suggested earlier, there are many categories of osteoporosis. They are classified as being primary or secondary. Primary osteoporosis includes both postmenopausal and age-related bone loss. Age-related loss affects both men and women as time goes on, but men lose bone much more slowly than do women. Postmenopausal osteoporosis, on the other hand, clearly affects only women and is very rapid. It is this type of osteoporosis that we will discuss here.

Secondary osteoporosis takes place when a specific disease or condition is responsible for skeletal bone erosion. Leukemia, hyperthyroidism (overactive thyroid), acromegaly (a problem stemming from the pituitary gland), rheumatoid arthritis, chronic lung disease and weightlessness (such as astronauts experience) will produce secondary osteoporosis in time.

Conditions that put certain women more at risk for osteoporosis include:

• *Genes and geography.* There are inherited characteristics for bone strength and weakness. Moreover, blacks are much less susceptible to osteoporosis than are Caucasian and Oriental women. Southern Europeans are more susceptible than their northern sisters.

• *Calcium deficiency.* Such deficiency may be due to inadequate calcium intake or to an inability to absorb calcium. This often occurs because of inadequate vitamin D intake.

• *Absent or inappropriate estrogen levels.* This is especially true in women who have lost their ovaries before the natural menopause.

• *Lack of regular, forceful exercise.*

• *Certain dietary aberrations.* Excess protein, caffeine, salt or alcohol may contribute to bone loss.

• *Tobacco.* Once again King Nicotine appears in the spoiler role.

• *Slight frame.* Thin women with small bones are at increased risk.

• *Childlessness.* Women who have never borne children seem to be at greater risk.

So if you are a short, thin, white, fair-complexioned lass approaching forty-five, and you sit on your can—indoors—all day, smoking, drinking alcohol and/or coffee, ingesting little or no calcium and failing to exercise—*watch out!* You are the perfect osteoporosis candidate.

The Diagnosis of Osteoporosis

Certainly our goal should be to prevent osteoporosis long, long before it becomes clinically evident, for osteoporosis is a silent thief, stealing bone for years before discovery. And restitution is just about impossible. We can barely catch the thief.

It therefore becomes important to anticipate the bone loss

and to concentrate our preventive efforts upon those women at risk. This may involve some overactive and generous treatment, even among women who are not going to develop menopausal osteoporosis, but treatment does not involve increased risk if handled carefully.

Regular office examinations should include annual measurement of standing or sitting height plus the assessment of back pain and discomfort. Loss of sitting or standing height—particularly in association with acute or chronic back discomfort—is often the first clinical clue to this disorder.

Most of the pain associated with collapsing vertebrae from osteoporosis will eventually disappear since these fractures are stable in character and the vertebrae will adjust to their new condition. With a subsequent fracture, new pain will appear. Some dull chronic mid-back pain that responds to bed rest may persist between fracture episodes, but continuing severe pain would be suspicious of another disorder. Therefore, in the diagnostic workup, assessment of back structure and spinal cord health is important.

LABORATORY TESTS

Routine laboratory testing is almost useless in the detection of PMPX osteoporisis. Blood and urine levels of calcium generally stay within normal limits during osteoporosis, as do most other markers of bone destruction. In fact, normal laboratory tests simply help rule out other diseases that can cause bone disorders. Under clinical investigation are a number of as-yet-unproven laboratory tests to detect early osteoporosis. Thus, measurement of a certain pituitary hormone (GnRH), serum estrogen levels, urinary excretion of a certain group of body by-products and numerous other laboratory procedures are all under study. But none is yet ready to be used.

IMAGING

There are several ways that picture-making can be useful, not only in making a diagnosis, but also in following the progression of osteoporosis. Imaging can also determine the bone's response to treatment. There are several types of imaging techniques:

• *X-rays.* Standard x-ray pictures of the skeleton will show collapsed, thin vertebrae along the backbone in advanced osteoporosis and will, of course, clearly show fractures. Yet x-rays cannot determine early loss of bone and so are not useful in the detection of osteoporosis.

• *Single photon absorptiometry (SPA).* This technique scans the wrist to see how much radiation from radioactive iodine is absorbed by the bones in that area. The radiation dose used is only 20 percent of that required for a chest x-ray. Although very precise, SPA measures primarily cortical bone, and so is not very useful in scanning the vertebrae or hips for trabecular bone loss.

• *Dual photon absorptiometry (DPA).* This technique involves the use of two photon beams of gadolinium. The rate at which these radioactive beams pass through the vertebrae or a hip bone will indicate, fairly accurately, the density of trabecular and cortical bone. As with SPA, there is little radiation exposure. Based on data supplied by DPA, it is possible to make fairly accurate predictions about future fracture risk.

• *Computerized axial tomography (CAT scan).* This technique, like DPA, measures radiation that passes through the bone. It has the distinct advantage of being able to separate trabecular from cortical bone. And it is very accurate. In a few areas of the United States, some special CAT scan equipment is individually designed for osteoporosis measurements. CAT scanning equipment is very expensive and usually hospital based. In addition, the radiation exposure in a CAT scan is significantly greater than in other imaging techniques.

• Ultrasound and magnetic resonance imaging are not at this time in clinical use for bone scanning.

All in all, the dual photon procedure is the most widely used and the most acceptable clinical measurement of bone density. But even *without* bone scanning of any sort, *without* laboratory procedures and *without* much clinical study at all, the diagnosis of osteoporosis can be made and treatment instituted. Moreover, our major strategy today in taming this disorder is to prevent it from ever taking place.

The Treatment of Osteoporosis

As you have already guessed, the ideal treatment of osteoporosis is prevention and that is our real goal. Once bone is lost to this silent thief, it is difficult—some say impossible—to replace. It may actually be, however, that newer programs can replace some of the lost bone. It is clear though, that customary present-day therapy can only arrest bone loss; it certainly cannot fix already fractured and collapsed vertebrae. So prevention is the goal.

Many factors are important in controlling osteoporosis—diet, calcium, exercise, vitamin D, fluoride, avoidance of tobacco and alcohol, and so on. But without estrogen, nothing else really works. So if prevention is the goal, estrogen is the road.

HORMONE REPLACEMENT THERAPY

HRT should be started as soon as internal production of estrogen diminishes to a symptomatic level (flushes, irregular menses, etc.) at the natural MPX or immediately after surgical removal of the ovaries in order to prevent osteoporosis. Of course, in every instance, there must be no valid contraindication to HRT. (See pages 59–60.)

Estrogen and progesterone should be given together for the following, already-stated reasons:

• Progesterone will protect the uterus against unilateral stimulation of estrogen, thus diminishing the risk of cancer of the endometrium.

• Many of us now believe progesterone has an equal protective effect against breast cancer. More believe it all the time but it is still not absolute.

• Estrogen retards bone loss, but it builds no new bone. Progesterone has been demonstrated to build new bone.

• By manipulating the dose of progesterone, it is usually possible to avoid menstruation in later years. Sixty-year-old patients are tired of carrying tampons in their purses.

HRT should be continued for at least ten years after the natural menopause, again to prevent osteoporosis. Many feel it should never be stopped—only reduced—as the years go by. Thus, if a woman sustains a surgical menopause at age thirty, for example, she should be supported by HRT for at least another thirty years. Unless something better comes along.

DIET

Most dietary habits involved in management of osteoporosis are noncontroversial, and most fall in line with your regular diet. (See pages 75–80.) The big controversy revolves around calcium—about which I could easily write a whole book. In general terms of diet, remember to avoid excesses of animal protein, caffeine, salt (any sodium, actually) and fiber.

Get as much dietary calcium as you can from food sources. Skim milk, low-fat yogurt, beans, cauliflower, broccoli, salmon, tofu and sardines are excellent sources, while most fruits, vegetables and cereals in your regular diet are good sources.

Don't drink more than two glasses of wine with your evening meal.

CALCIUM

For some time it was felt that adequate calcium intake alone could prevent osteoporosis. This is no longer a tenable theory. And rightly so. It is true that our average calcium intake is insufficient for our needs, but increased consumption alone is not enough.

American women take in about 650 mg of calcium daily. As you know, that isn't enough to maintain your daily calcium balance of 800 mg. Remember, that is 800 mg of pure calcium. The most common calcium supplement (calcium carbonate) is *less than* half calcium.

Most MPX women should have at least 1000 mg calcium daily—one way or another. Too much calcium is as bad as too little. Don't overdose.

Calcium levels in blood and other tissues must be kept constant. This regulation is managed by the parathyroid and thyroid glands. The thyroid gland secretes the hormone calcitonin, which is responsible for putting calcium back in bones when it's not needed for other bodily processes. However, low levels of calcitonin take calcium from bone to replace calcium not obtained from the diet. More on calcitonin later. The parathyroid glands, through their hormones, further fine-tune calcium blood levels.

The 1000–1500 mg suggested calcium intake does not increase your risk of calcium kidney stones or affect your medication for heart disease and high blood pressure (hypertension). In fact, it is becoming increasingly clear that an adequate dietary calcium intake protects against hypertension.

As you already know, estrogen has a protective effect upon bone and facilitates the absorption of calcium, thereby reducing its excretion via the kidneys.

So, what should your calcium program consist of?

• Eat a proper diet and you will get at least 650 mg calcium daily.

• Take about 400–500 mg more of pure calcium as a supplement. Two Tums, for instance, deliver 1000 mg of calcium carbonate (400 mg of calcium). Calcium carbonate (there are many other kinds of calcium supplements on the market) may be taken alone or with meals. Its only side effect may be constipation. Remember, don't overdose. More is not better.

• Include calcium citrate in your diet. Calcium citrate is becoming available on the market, both as a tablet and in certain fruit juices. It is absorbed more by the body more readily than any other form of calcium. Read labels for amounts and the available pure calcium.

• For maximum benefit, begin calcium supplementation early on. Remember, women begin to lose bone in their thirties due to inadequate calcium intake.

EXERCISE

Although there is no single, cleanly structured study that would prove the value of exercise in osteoporosis management, there is certainly a great deal of peripheral evidence. And, as you are aware, a regular exercise program has significant, progressive and prolonged value in your postmenopausal years.

If possible, it is important to build bone mass through diet and exercise before the menopause. Clear evidence indicates bone mass responds to repeated challenge. Thus, a tennis player may have as much as a 30 percent increase in bone mass in the racquet-holding arm! Other athletes show similar bone-growth responses. Conversely, bones rapidly demineralize in weightless individuals (such as astronauts).

As aging progresses and as falls become more ominous and more common, exercise is protective for two reasons: first, stability is improved and so falls are less likely to take place, and second, the increased mobility generated by regular exercise helps you "roll into" a fall and cushion its effect.

Incidentally, your home environment should eliminate as many "fall" traps as possible. Throw rugs, polished floors, loose steps and any other potentially dangerous articles should be banished.

OTHER FACTORS IN OSTEOPOROSIS CONTROL

VITAMIN D. This essential vitamin has several important roles in bone metabolism. It supports calcium absorption, slows calcium loss and promotes maintenance of the bone mass. Many food products (milk, for instance) have vitamin D added. Read the labels.

Vitamin D supplements are not necessary for women who

are exposed to sunlight year-round. However, experts are now advising us to stay out of the sun because of the recent fearsome rise in a certain deadly type of skin cancer (melanoma). This cancer increase is attributed to overexposure to the heavier doses of ultraviolet rays now able to penetrate earth's polluted atmosphere.

Your daily intake of vitamin D need not exceed 600–800 international units. Overdosing with D can be very dangerous and will not help retain bone mass.

FLUORIDES. A very popular topic today. Fluorides will, in sufficient amounts, help build new bone, particularly trabecular bone. Whether they prevent bone loss is not clear. Therefore, the use of fluorides in osteoporosis must be considered experimental at this time.

If fluorides are used to treat osteoporosis, adequate amounts of calcium and vitamin D must also be given concurrently. Otherwise, serious bone disorders may follow.

Most urban water supplies in the United States now contain fluoride in varying amounts, mainly for prophylaxis (preventive benefits) against dental decay. The amount is very small, and its value in preventing osteoporosis at these levels is unknown.

Side effects of high fluoride dosage, such as leg cramps and skin rashes, occur in half the patients under study. The National Institutes of Health have several large-scale ongoing studies right now.

Don't try to get sodium fluoride on your own—yet.

CALCITONIN. Another hot item. You already know that calcitonin is secreted by the thyroid gland and that when the level of calcitonin circulating throughout the body decreases, it is a very important trigger in bone loss. Calcitonin has been used experimentally and is now FDA-approved for use in treating osteoporosis. However:

- It is very expensive and has to be given by injection or by nasal spray daily.

- There are often marked side effects of calcitonin administration.

- Calcitonin will not build new bone; it only slows the loss of old bone.

- Therapy with this drug should be reserved for severe osteoporosis that fails to respond to conventional lines of treatment.

- It is worth noting that both birth control pills and oral estrogens increase natural calcitonin levels.

DYAZIDE THERAPY. Dyazides, which are a group of diuretic (fluid control) medications, are now being used as a second-line treatment source for osteoporosis. These drugs promote the loss of water through the kidneys, and at the same time promote reabsorption of calcium, thus decreasing urinary calcium loss. There are, as always, potent side effects from dyazides, so they must be used with caution and only in patients with nonresponding osteoporosis.

Other treatments are in use here and there to manage osteoporosis. Testosterone, for instance—the hormone that athletes use to build bone and muscle mass—is clearly a positive force in building bone. It must, however, be balanced with estrogen and given with great care.

Experimental Osteoporosis Programs

Most osteoporosis studies involve attempts to build new bone or remodel existing bone structures. For instance, the use of calcitonin and oral phosphates to stimulate parathyroid activity and thus bone retention is one approach being studied at this time.

As an extension of the above experiments, a group of scientists are following up a cycle of parathyroid and phosphates with an additional two weeks of Didronel (etidronate disodium). This cycle of medication is repeated at regular intervals and the rate of new bone growth is very encouraging.

Human parathyroid hormone (HPTH), when administered along with a certain type of vitamin D, has been shown (in an experimental study group) to promote new bone growth. The study is continuing.

It is known that electrical field activity accelerates fracture healing. This technique is now being tried experimentally as a method of promoting new bone growth.

Other possible cures are too far down the line to even report upon. And all of a sudden, from a totally unexpected and unrelated source, the perfect treatment may appear. If you don't believe that's possible, read the story of the discovery of penicillin.

◄§ Pause and Reflect

Salmon is not only a good source of omega-3 fatty acids (see page 83), it is also rich in calcitonin. So, for that matter, are eels and lizards!

Most women who develop gouty arthritis (a condition in which crystalized substances are deposited within joint cavities, causing stiffness and pain) develop it after the menopause. Women receiving HRT, however, are apparently protected from gout and in one recent study, no woman on HRT could be found with the disorder.

Psychotropic drugs (tranquilizers) have been implicated in hip fractures among older women. With certain of these agents, the risk was increased up to 80 percent! Why? Most likely—although not certainly—because they caused increased instability and thus greater tendency to fall.

Investigators are attempting to manufacture the proteins responsible for bone healing in fractures. They would then harvest such proteins and use them to promote new bone growth.

Although exercise early on in life is very important in providing superior bone mass going into the menopause, can exercise be overdone? How do athletes fare in the MPX?

Many studies show that the average high school and college athlete does very well in the MPX, at least as well as her nonathletic counterpart. However, those women involved in strenuous, continued athletic competition—sufficient to induce amenorrhea and estrogen insufficiency—sustained bone loss of a significant degree in their vertebrae. What this will produce in later years is not yet known.

Compared to currently married menopausal women, single, never-married women are over twice as likely to be hospitalized with a fractured hip, while divorced or widowed women are 1.7 times more likely to be hospitalized.

Calcium from whole milk, chocolate milk, yogurt, imitation milk, and pure calcium carbonate are all absorbed equally well.

CHAPTER TEN

Breasts and the Menopausal Woman

It is strange and disturbing that a body part as lionized, talked about, photographed, painted, almost venerated, is as poorly understood insofar as disorders are concerned, as the female breasts.

For example, cancer of the breast remains almost an enigma, while cancer of the lung is completely understood; the cause, the cure and the prevention are totally clear to us. Sadly, this cancer of the lung has overtaken cancer of the breast as the greatest malignant killer of women. This is not because breast cancer is decreasing, which it is not, but because lung cancer is increasing. This increase, of course, is based upon the increased number of women who began smoking at the end of World War II.

At any rate, we are just now beginning to understand the individual growth characteristics of breast cancer. It continues at the same occurrence rate or may gradually be increasing, and our treatment is no better—only slightly more humane and less mutilating.

Breast Physiology and Anatomy

In each female human breast, there are usually eighteen separate lobes. Each lobe contains glands that will secrete milk after the woman gives birth to a child, and ducts that will lead the milk to each nipple. Therefore, each nipple has eighteen separate ducts leading to it. This glandular and duct system is supported in a fibro-fatty network which holds everything in place. That, then, is the very basic architecture of each breast.

At the *thenarche,* which usually takes place from the ninth to eleventh year of childhood, the female breast tissue (which has been dormant) comes under the stimulation of a number of hormones—mainly estrogen, progesterone and human growth hormone. These substances promote growth and development of the breast, so that it becomes a mature organ capable of producing milk upon stimulation after obstetrical delivery.

Breasts also respond to other hormones. For instance, a pituitary hormone called *prolactin* is necessary for normal milk production. Incidentally, it also prevents menstruation. Thus, when a pituitary tumor of a certain type is present, excess prolactin is secreted and, even when the woman is in a nonpregnant state, there will be secretion from the nipples (not milk, however) and absence of menstruation. This disorder is easily diagnosed but not so easily treated.

Other hormones secreted by the thyroid and adrenal glands affect breast growth and development, and another pituitary hormone, *oxytocin,* is responsible for the beginning of milk ejection during late labor and following delivery.

Of all these hormones, estrogen and progesterone have far and away the greatest effect on breast tissue. Estrogen is necessary for growth and development of the glandular tissue and progesterone is necessary for the maturation of many aspects of these tissues. As we move along in the study of breast disorders, we will see what effect these two hormones may or may not have.

Breast Disorders

Although there are many problems that can occur in breast tissue, ranging from simple infection during nursing all the way to cancer, there are three that occupy most of physicians' time and attention.

First, *cystic mastitis:* This is a very common disorder that results from the normal influence of estrogen and progesterone on the breast's glandular and duct structure. Usually it begins with unexplained duct obstruction, and as secretions back up behind the obstruction, tense, swollen gland tissue ensues. That in turn produces inflammation and tenderness. The end result is fibrosis, or scarring of local areas of breast tissue. Clinically, doctors can detect this condition when the breast tissue feels nodular and irregular in outline and has some firm areas of swelling and tenderness. Interestingly enough, as we will see later on, cystic mastitis tends to be less likely to occur in women who have been on oral contraceptives for a reasonably long period of time.

Cystic mastitis generally is characterized by breast pain, which may be intermittent in nature, may be worst just prior to periods and may be accompanied by nipple discharge. For some unknown reason, caffeine consumption apparently increases the irritation and pain of cystic mastitis. Whether cystic mastitis leads on to cancer or predisposes women to cancer is a hotly debated item. The consensus of present day thought is that it does not. Treatment consists of various hormone programs and caffeine restriction.

The second disorder is called *fibroadenoma.* Usually this

condition develops in young women, but it also may occur at the perimenopause and even postmenopausally if hormone replacement therapy, particularly unopposed estrogen replacement therapy, is employed. Fibroadenomas, which are small, firm tumors present in the gland substance of one or more lobes, are caused by the *unilateral* stimulation of estrogen at any time in reproductive life. The problem is found more commonly in youngsters and in perimenopausal women because these individuals are usually not ovulating and thus not producing progesterone.

Fibroadenomas are benign tumors that may vary in size during menstrual cycles but will not disappear completely. They usually can be clearly defined by mammography. Generally no treatment is necessary, unless they cannot be clearly distinguished from breast cancer, at which time excision biopsy (complete removal of the growth at biopsy) is indicated.

The third breast disorder is *hyperplasia* (overgrowth) of gland and duct epithelium (lining cells). In this disorder, excess cells are formed in the surface layer of the milk-producing glands and ducts. This condition, which is very difficult to diagnose, is also apparently related to unilateral or unopposed estrogen stimulation. Both glandular and ductal hyperplasia are usually found when biopsies are performed for other, more obvious abnormalities in breast tissue. Symptoms are generally slight, and usually include a bloody discharge from the nipples. Very little or nothing can be felt in these cases. The only treatment is the administration of progesterone. The relationship of this condition to breast cancer is uncertain.

Cancer of the Breast

The enormity of this problem cannot be overstated. Although cancer of the lung has now supplanted breast cancer as the leading cause of malignant death among women in this country, it is only because cancer of the lung has been increasing regularly over the years. Mortality from cancer of the breast is more or less the same as it was thirty years ago, with some very early indications of a change in that pattern. From the press and television you are already painfully aware that breast cancer will develop in one in every eleven women in this country, and the vast majority of those women will eventually die from this condition. It was expected that over 125,000 women would develop cancer of the breast in 1988 and the solution to this problem is nowhere in sight.

Cancer of the breast rarely occurs before women reach age twenty-five and is most commonly a disease of the perimenopausal and menopausal years. Its rate of spread, its treatment and the end results are variable depending upon the woman's age when the tumor first develops.

Recent understanding of the life history of breast cancer has changed our treatment of this disorder to a great degree. Originally, the theory of breast cancer disease was that it began in the breast tissue, spreading much later to the lymph glands in the armpits, and then traveling elsewhere in the body. It is now understood that the disease at a very early stage becomes a systemic disease. Thus, surgery that is local and severely mutilating is not as helpful in the management of the disease as is local removal of the tumor area and systemic treatment. This has yielded slightly better results with less body mutilation.

WHO IS AT GREATEST RISK FOR DEVELOPING
BREAST CANCER?

The following factors determine who is most likely to develop
breast cancer:

  • *Family history.* Women whose family history includes female relatives who have had breast cancer have a significantly greater risk, particularly if these relatives are on the
  maternal side, and particularly if their breast cancer developed earlier in life (before the menopause).

  • *Age at menopause.* The later the menopause begins, the
  greater the risk of developing breast cancer. This may be
  related to prolonged unopposed estrogen production after
  ovulation ceases.

  • *Pregnancy.* Pregnancy exerts, probably through hormonal
  patterns, a protective influence against the development of
  breast cancer. The earlier the pregnancies occur, the greater
  the protection. Thus, women who have never borne children
  are at a greater risk for breast cancer.

  • *Ovarian activity.* Women with prolonged anovulatory cycles (periods of time during which ovulation does not occur),
  that is, who are exposed to unopposed estrogen over the
  years, are at greater risk.

  • *Nutrition.* Women who are obese, women who are diabetic and women who are on a high-cholesterol diet are more
  susceptible to breast cancer. This again is related to the production and storage (in fat) of unopposed estrogen. Also on a
  nutritional basis, there is now evidence that alcohol consumption increases the risk of breast cancer. It is important to point
  out here that the data upon which this conclusion is based is

recent and not clearly established. However, this is something that bears further study.

• *Ethnic background.* It is clear that some ethnic groups are at greater risk of developing breast cancer. Thus, North American and Western European women are at significantly greater risk than are Japanese, black and Indian women. Moreover, women in an upper socioeconomic level are at greater risk. This may be related to many factors that are not directly involved with social background.

• *Previous breast cancer in one of the breasts.* This clearly increases the risk of recurrence in both breasts. There is now considerable controversy among experts in the field, some suggesting that after cancerous breast tissue is removed, removal of the other breast (along with plastic reconstruction of both breasts) may be a wise procedure. More on this later.

• *Other factors.* Previous multiple chest x-rays; marital status; country versus city living and so forth also play some role in the genesis of this disorder.

The Diagnosis of Breast Cancer

Many techniques have been employed in order to facilitate and speed up the diagnosis of breast cancer. It is very clear that the earlier the diagnosis is made, the more successful treatment will be, and the greater the quality of life in the survivor. There are three basic methods of diagnosis.

BREAST SELF-EXAMINATION

Although considered an anachronism by many scientists, it still remains the most productive method of detecting breast cancer today: 90 percent of all breast cancers are discovered by breast self-examination. It has been shown that women who are unskilled at breast self-examination cannot detect a tumor until it is at least *twice* the size of a tumor that a more skilled woman could identify. The technique is explained in many of the free pamphlets published and distributed widely by the American Cancer Society. (Write to the American Cancer Society, 90 Park Avenue, New York, NY 10016, and they will be happy to send you an outline.) In addition, many physicians have pamphlets in their offices describing the technique for breast self-examination and breast cancer detection centers teach and encourage this form of examination.

In many instances, husbands become skilled supplemental breast examiners, and they should be encouraged to do this regardless of what sexual overtones can be read into it. I advise you to learn breast self-examination. During the first year of self-examination your breasts may feel lumpy, irregular and filled with disease, but you will eventually come to know the topography and architecture of your breasts very well.

PHYSICIAN BREAST EXAMINATION

Regular palpation of breast tissue by your physician should be a part of your annual examination. Under certain circumstances, more frequent examinations are clearly indicated. Your physician's examination may be different from your own examination, but the same structural abnormalities are being sought after. You should be willing, indeed anxious, to have your physician examine your breasts, and he or she should be equally anxious to do so for you. Again, early de-

tection is vitally important and you and your physician together can do a better job than either one alone. Persistent
breast masses should be identified and diagnosed to every-
body's satisfaction.

IMAGING TECHNIQUES

These diagnostic procedures are far and away the most important methods available today in making an early diagnosis of
breast cancer. The techniques used today include mammography, ultrasound, and magnetic resonance imaging.

MAMMOGRAPHY. Of all the imaging techniques, nothing at this
time approaches the mammogram in its efficiency in deter-
mining the presence or absence of a breast lesions and identi-
fying their malignant or nonmalignant characters. Here are
some very salient points about mammography:

   • Although not 100 percent successful in finding breast cancer, mammography has the lowest failure rate of any known
   technique today. It will often detect a tumor as many as two
   or more years before it could have been felt either by the
   woman or her physician.

   • All mammograms involve the use of x-rays. Mammogram
   exposure rates, insofar as radiation risks are concerned, are
   minimal, however. Assuming a patient had twenty mammograms in a lifetime, her radiation exposure risks in terms of
   developing cancer would be equivalent to smoking *four* or
   five cigarettes in a *lifetime.* This would appear to be a very
   acceptable risk.

   • Mammogram screening clinics are springing up every-
   where in the United States. Screening mammograms are
   done in every kind of setting—x-ray offices, doctors' offices,

mobile clinics, shopping malls—anywhere a certified techni-
cian with the proper equipment can set up shop. They are
taken as a routine age-based screen and are not taken when
disease is present or suspected. Under those circumstances a
mammogram is diagnostic and is performed at a radiology
clinic only. Screening clinics are increasing the availability of
this technique and, by and large, decreasing the cost. As an
example, there are four mammographic screening clinics in
the Little Rock area. These clinics, which generally operate
on a walk-in basis, charge $65 for a mammogram and an
explanation of breast self-examination. In some places, a
mammogram can cost up to $300, but competition is rapidly
eliminating such elitist institutions. Mammograms should be
read by certified radiologists, preferably ones who have received added training in the interpretation of mammograms.
This is true even for screening mammograms.

• Mammograms are most useful among women who are in
the age groups most likely to develop breast cancer. This
disease almost never occurs before age twenty-five, and its
frequency of occurrence diminishes among women in their
sixties and seventies. Several associations have recommended
that women without known breast disease and with no
known family history of breast disease should have a screening mammogram at age thirty-five, then one every two years
between forty and fifty, and then one every year once they
reach their fifties and sixties. This recommendation will undoubtedly change in the next few years as more women in
their forties undergo annual rather than biennial screening.
(This projection is based on studies that reveal a greater survival rate of women in this age group who have had regular
annual mammograms.) In families with a strong breast cancer
history, particularly if cancer has developed before the menopause in close family relatives, the frequency at which mam-

mograms are obtained will vary somewhat. Your physician will determine what's best for you.

ULTRASOUND IMAGING. This very safe, noninvasive method of imaging has been applied to examinations of the breast. At the present time, ultrasound is not used as a screening technique, but instead is used in cases where routine mammographic screening has revealed breast tissue that is thick or difficult to penetrate clearly by mammography. Such tissue needs further, localized study. Ultrasound procedures are not generally used then in screening clinics, but only where a screening mammogram has revealed a disorder or where an inadequate screening examination requires further delineation or study. Under these circumstances, ultrasound studies are performed in a radiology clinic, and a radiologist is generally present to help in localizing and diagnosing particular areas of the breast in question. It may well be that three-dimensional ultrasound examination will be the procedure of choice in the future insofar as breast screening is concerned. For the present, however, that is not the case.

MAGNETIC RESONANCE IMAGING (MRI). This fantastic—but very expensive—imaging procedure is now available at most medical centers throughout the United States. In Little Rock there are now three such establishments. As with ultrasound, magnetic resonance imaging involves no radiation whatsoever and poses no risk to the patient submitting to it. MRI may be the wave of the future in terms of early detection of breast malignancies, but at the present time, its expense and unavailability make it an unusual screening technique.

THERMOGRAPHY AND TRANSILLUMINATION. These procedures involve the radiation of heat from breast tissue or the transillumination of light through it. Tumors radiate more heat and will not transilluminate light. At this time, neither appears to be terribly accurate, even for minor screening techniques. Neither is recommended at this time.

The Treatment of Breast Cancer

This is a very complicated and complex subject that we cannot begin to cover in this menopause handbook. Basically, the treatment will vary significantly depending on whether the patient is premenopausal or postmenopausal and whether or not the lymph nodes in the armpits test positive for cancer cells. Again, there appears to be less emphasis today on radical local surgery and more upon local excision of tumor mass and more generalized body treatment with radiation and/or chemotherapy. Should you, God forbid, be diagnosed as having a breast malignancy, you should consult two competent breast surgeons before submitting to any therapy.

HRT and Breast Cancer

As you already know, hormone replacement therapy involving proper combinations of estrogen and progesterone does not cause cancer of the endometrium, and in fact protects the endometrium against the development of malignancies. Since breast tissue contains target cells affected by estrogen and progesterone, won't the combination of estrogen and progesterone protect this tissue against the ultimate development of breast cancer? Although there is still considerable argument among investigative scientists in this regard, it is becoming clear that estrogen and progesterone (progestin) given in proper combinations will protect the breasts against the development of cancer. The evidence is as follows:

• Women who have been on long-term oral contraceptives (which are a combination of synthetic estrogen and progestins) have been conclusively shown to have less risk of breast cancer than women who have not taken oral contraceptives. A thorough review of all of the literature on oral contraceptives refutes the view that they increase the risk of breast cancer.

• Women who develop breast cancer and formerly used birth control pills have a greater overall survival rate than those breast cancer patients who never used birth control pills.

• The largest studies accumulated to date on the use of HRT in menopausal and postmenopausal women clearly show that the breast is protected against cancer by the use of combined estrogen and progesterone replacement therapy. The use of estrogen alone appears to be nonprotective but has not clearly been perceived to be dangerous.

• When progestational agents are experimentally added to cultures of human breast cancer cells, the multiplication of cancer cells is inhibited.

Thus, it is evident that in the absence of an existing breast cancer, appropriately given hormone replacement therapy will protect the human female breasts against the development of cancer. It is becoming clear, however, that progestin compounds must be included in such HRT therapy.

HRT Following Breast Cancer

For a number of reasons, it has become appropriate to consider the institution of hormone replacement therapy in women who have undergone adequate therapy for cancer of the breast. This is particularly true in young women who have had breast cancer and who are having significant menopausal problems. Severe flushes, depression and vaginal atrophy with painful intercourse are examples.

Since many breast cancers are "estrogen dependent" and thus grow more readily in its presence, hormone replacement therapy can be considered only in cases where the breast tumor was discovered very early and when there has been evidence of complete arrest for at least five years. Although there is not a large body of research available in this area, more and more data supporting HRT after breast cancer are accumulated as each year goes by. Research is limited by the risks of malpractice, the dogmas of prior teaching authorities and prior theories, and by clearly understandable patient fears. Yet many patients, having been thoroughly informed about the risks and benefits of hormonal replacement therapy following five years of cancer arrest, are now accepting HRT. The safety of such programs cannot, of course, be documented for many years to come.

Let me end this disheartening section on breast cancer with what I feel is a great coming breakthrough in the treatment of all cancers.

Immunologists, using monoclonal antibody technology (which is too complex to explain and not necessary to explain for our needs anyway), can now make immune proteins for specific cancers. These can then be "radiolabeled" with minute amounts of radioactivity. Injected into the blood stream, these immune antibodies attach at once to any such cancer cells in the body. Screening the body now will identify if cancer is present and give a clear picture of its extent and/or spread. Thus, if breast cancer antibodies are injected and there are no breast cancer cells present, screening of the breast tissue for radioactivity will reveal none and so the test will be negative. If, on the other hand, a breast cancer exists, it will be found, no matter how small, and screening will tell its extent and location clearly, and any spread will be visualized as well—a marvelous diagnostic tool. But there is more.

Using the same monoclonal antibodies—this time made highly radioactive—we can thus inject a cancer killer that will go directly to the tumor cells no matter where they are, grab hold and go nowhere else!

There is still much to be done, but investigators feel this technique will be in use in this century.

◄§ *Pause and Reflect*

As a part of sex-change therapy, genetic-true males who are being converted into females are given large doses of estrogen that will produce enlargement of the breasts. No progesterone or progestins are given. There are now *two* reported cases of breast cancer among such genetic males receiving estrogen therapy. This does not speak well for the way breast tissue responds to unopposed estrogen.

Women whose breasts have been augmented by surgical procedures (implanted prosthetic devices) can still be studied properly by routine mammographic examinations. Such examinations are, however, much more difficult to interpret.

———————

Some evidence exists that women who have pacemakers inserted in the chest wall should undergo more frequent mammographic examinations. One study has revealed a threefold increase in breast cancer on the side in which a pacemaker has been implanted. Although this particular subject might now be debated, it still should not be overlooked.

———————

If every woman in the United States between the ages of fifty and seventy-five had a mammogram at an average cost of $80, the annual bill would be $3.3 billion. Since the total health care cost in the United States exceeds $400 billion a year, and since breast cancer one of the leading causes of death among American women, it appears that routine mammography screening might save insurance companies a great deal of money and American women a great deal of grief. Most insurance companies, however, do not hold this view.

———————

In a recent study conducted in Scotland, 12,000 women were given small-group lectures on breast self-examination. Prior to the instruction, 11% of these women practiced breast self-examination. A year later, only 13% of these women practiced the self-examinations.

Much worse than that, only 11% of physicians in the United States contacted in one study recommended regular mammographic examinations as outlined by the American Cancer Society, the American College of Obstetricians and Gynecologists, and the American College of Surgeons. Of those physicians interviewed, 39% said mammograms cost too much, 29% said they were unnecessary for women without any symptoms and 25% said the patients were exposed to too much radiation. So patient compliance is one part of the problem, but physician leadership is an even greater one and probably the more disturbing of the two.

CHAPTER ELEVEN

Aging

Let's face it: Aging, like death and taxes, is inexorable, inevitable and unavoidable. And though we understand very little about death or taxes, we are making some headway in our understanding of aging. Let's look at what we know. And let's look at the good news about what we can expect on the positive side!

There are a bunch of us growing old. That's true. But we are doing it better and doing it longer. During Caesar's heyday in Rome, life expectancy was around twenty-five years. At the turn of this century, it was forty years. Today, a sixty-five-year-old woman can plan on at least another twenty years of life, and a newborn female can expect to live well into her middle or late eighties.

Thus the ranks of Master Citizens are mushrooming. A gynecologist may well be spending 75 percent of all office time seeing women over age sixty-five by the time this century elapses. By that time one person in seven will be over sixty-five.

Although during this century we have gained more life expectancy than we have in the preceding 5,000 years, doctors have not kept up with our medical understanding of this population of people. Until recently, studies of aging have been performed primarily upon residents of nursing homes. This is not a healthy group of aging people, and thus conclusions drawn from such studies have clearly been inadequate and incorrect. Only recently have we begun to collect reliable data on aging in a healthy population. The results are quite astounding.

The medical profession, working with the limited available information on aging, has not helped the problem much. Too often doctors have lumped their senior citizens together as a bunch of stupid, cranky, uncooperative old fools. Moreover, medical schools are only now beginning to incorporate significant geriatric training into their curricula so that the newly graduated doctors will understand the problems and concerns of this large segment of their practices. Until recently, medical schools ignored this part of the population.

How We Age

Remember that aging is an inevitable process that we are just beginning to understand. And regardless of how much we understand of aging and how successful we may become in slowing it down, it still chips away at us all and will some day work its final will upon each and every one of us. With that heartening introduction, here's some of what we know about aging.

Aging changes begin slowly in the thirties (remember what you read about the start of bone loss) and pick up after the menopause, accelerating thereafter.

Fundamental to the aging process is a decrease in the body's ability to adapt to stress, and consequently an increase in the body's vulnerability to damage. A very simple example of this fact would be the Master Citizen's response to influenza; it's usually a mild disorder of young people, but it's a potential killer of older people. The altered physiology behind the aging body's loss of adaptibility is not yet known.

A major source of continued stress appears to be substances and activities that chronically irritate various body surfaces, such as the skin, intestinal tract, lungs, genitourinary tract and so on. Add to this the fact that cell division becomes less perfect as time goes by (and irritants speed up the rate of cell division), and imperfect cell division sets the stage for malignant changes, which destroy one-third to one-half of all senior citizens.

In women (as you are now well aware) the absence of estrogen that accompanies aging signals a rapid increase in bone loss, arteriosclerosis, and sexual tissue atrophy.

As aging progresses, it appears that the circulating levels of certain protective white blood cells (lymphocytes) decrease. This may help explain why immunizations are more difficult to achieve and maintain in the older population. Also, autoimmune antibodies (antibodies against one's own body) appear more frequently as aging continues. If these findings are thoroughly confirmed, it would account for many destructive processes in the elderly, particularly various forms of arthritis.

These basic facts about aging are greatly altered by what happens during our lives and by our lifestyles. More on that in a minute.

The Effects of Aging on Certain Body Systems

Listed below are ways specific parts of your body and certain bodily functions react to the aging process.

THE BRAIN

The intellectual capacities of a normal brain remain stable until we reach at least seventy. Although memory chips and cognitive chips are disappearing at the rate of 100,000 or so each day after age forty, there is a tremendous untapped reservoir of these "Golgi" (think cells) chips in brain storage, so that their loss is not deeply felt. Thus the intellectual capacities go on as always into the seventies. New research establishes quite clearly that these remaining untapped brain chips can actually be *brought on line* and utilized. That means we can rejoice in the continued *expansion* of our brainpower by simply reprogramming our software! All this, of course, can take place only in a healthy aging brain, where neurological disease has not taken an irreversible toll.

THE SKELETON

As you know, bone loss begins in the thirties, accelerates rapidly during the years just after menopause, then continues at a slower pace thereafter. Fractures appear in the sixty- to eighty-year age group with nonhealing being the usual course of events. You are aware of the factors accelerating this common crippling disorder, osteoporosis.

HEART AND LUNGS

High blood pressure is more likely to be present along with arteriosclerosis, and cardiac output in general is decreased. Lung expansion decreases, thus limiting the ability to consume oxygen and decreasing aerobic reserve. These factors increase the risk of strokes and heart attacks.

BLOOD

The composition of the blood is little changed as the years go by. Total blood counts of both red and white cells (except perhaps for lymphocytes—see above) should be at the same levels as always. The bone marrow maintains its ability to replace and rebuild blood levels rapidly. Thus, anemia in a ninety-year-old woman should be thoroughly investigated since it generally signifies hidden blood loss rather than iron deficiency.

METABOLISM

It is commonly accepted by doctors that as their patients age, the patients lose their ability to metabolize sugar. Thus age-onset diabetes is not an unexpected problem in the oldster. However, it now appears that sugar tolerance studies for Master Citizens are undoubtedly incorrect and too rigid, thus consigning innocent victims to the diabetes enclave. Moreover, the apparently age-related decline in ability to metabolize sugar often can be reversed by an increase in physical activity.

In other metabolic areas, the number of calories required to maintain body weight decreases as time goes on. Therefore, if caloric intake doesn't decline and activity levels remain the same, body weight will increase. In that regard I am not telling you anything you didn't know. But now new insurance tables come to the rescue! Guess what. The old tables were all too strict. We Masters should all weigh about 10–15 pounds *more* than formerly advocated. Hallelujah!

MUSCLE MASS

As time goes by, muscle mass and strength tend to decline. This may be due to tissue aging or to the absence of male or male-like hormones. However, the weight of evidence reveals that *lack of physical activity* is the greatest thief of muscle. Thus, at almost any age, physical activity will rebuild muscle.

SEXUAL ORGANS

This has been completely covered elsewhere (page 42). Once ovarian activity ceases, women begin to have atrophy of the vulva and vagina, loss of lubrication, orgasmic delay or absence, loss of sexual fantasies and diminished sexual drive.

SKIN

Your wraparound is vastly affected by any number of internal and external factors. Sunlight exposure, weight gain and loss, diet, smoking and alcohol and many other factors enter into what you have to look at each morning in the mirror. Generally, the skin ages more rapidly than other systems when it is subject to prolonged irritation. When estrogen is absent, skin collagen (supportive tissues) regularly disappears and the wrinkling rate accelerates. The greatest skin damage is probably done by sunlight; and the thinning atmosphere, combined with our sun worship, poses for us a dangerous epidemic of fatal skin cancer (melanoma). For those of you with delicate skin, remember, the porcelain look is "in." Even if sun exposure has never bothered your skin, minimize your cancer risk by staying out of the sun.

TEETH

Although tooth cavitation (the development of cavities) usually decreases at this time, bone erosion will often loosen teeth so that they fall out. Changes in occlusion (the way teeth fit together when the jaws are closed), caused by bone and tooth loss, also often induce gum disease and, in the past, the price was "teeth in a cup." Changing hygiene practices and modern orthodontics have reversed these unpleasant oral problems.

The Psychology of Aging

We have had a wealth of theory surrounding a poverty of solutions regarding the psychology of aging. Yet those involved in the mental health care of Master Citizens are beginning to recognize the following baseline psychological principles:

· Older people are generally more intelligent and worldly than those attempting to manage them. They have command, by and large, of a much greater vocabulary and have a more catholic and profound outlook on life. The fact that they may not want to take the time to share it with a neophyte does not mean it is not there. This is, of course, not always true. A fool at thirty will probably be a fool at sixty-five. (But a lot of fools are gone by sixty-five.)

· Most Master Citizens are proud and independent. They abhor disrespectful treatment and respond to it in kind.

Being designated by a case number, or worse still, by a first name, will draw the contempt it begs. It is worth noting that 70 percent of twenty- to twenty-five-year-olds interviewed stated that senior citizens should be cared for in their children's homes, while only 16 percent of the senior citizens agreed!

• The greatest crises that Master Citizens face are not challenges (career changes, for example) but losses due to death and separation as well as losses of physical function. These are the problems they most certainly and inevitably have to deal with.

Master Citizens, then, wish to preserve their identity and have the liberty to be their "eccentric" selves, but need compassionate, nonpatronizing help in managing the gradual loss of all things they hold dear.

Lifestyles for the Long Haul

Here are some ideas to help prepare you for a superb winter harvest: To begin with, nowhere else does the edict "use it or lose it" apply more directly. You have seen that many of the body systems once believed to crumble away with age are, in fact, able to grow and function much later in life. Thus, using, prodding and pushing your brain, muscles and cardiovascular system will not only maintain the status quo, but will cause your body to continuously respond by further growth.

Eat properly in accordance with the advice you have been given. Keep your caloric intake adjusted to your exercise demands. Take extra calcium and iron till you no longer make estrogen. If you are on hormone replacement therapy, continue calcium supplements.

Exercise regularly within the guidelines that have been laid out for you. Avoid excessive, high-impact exercise. Try to make exercise constructive, exciting and rewarding. Boring exercise will not last except in the most driven few.

Don't smoke—ever. Drink alcohol sparingly, and if you are hypertensive (have high blood pressure), not at all.

If you have an acceptable sexual outlet, do everything you can to keep an active sexual life going. HRT with local supplements will create the atmosphere.

Chances are you have been frying your skin for years and it is now years older than you. Wear protective clothing when you are in sunlight, and avoid tanning booths. If you must be in the sunlight, use the strongest filter cream you can get. If you're concerned about wrinkles, the only local application that may help wrinkles is Retin-A. Recent short-term studies suggest that this cream may help obliterate some wrinkles and may reverse some abnormal skin changes (photoaging). The studies are short-term as yet, the cream is expensive, and many people (90 percent) develop rashes, some severe, during therapy. The instructions *must be followed to the letter.* HRT has been shown to help rebuild thinning skin.

In preparation for the postmenopausal years—just as in preparation for early years—it is important to be prepared for the things that will come forward to challenge your coping abilities. We will age, we will see loved ones fall away, we will experience loneliness and, yes, depression at times. Learning to cope with these different problems before they are upon us is important. Many communities have groups that can help here. Try your AARP (American Association of Retired Persons). Remember: stay involved.

Avoid as many medications as you can. By virtue of your simply following the above rules, most medication will not be needed. Be sure you understand clearly what the reasoning behind your medication is, what its side effects may be and what other medications or foods may react unfavorably with it. Take what medicine you must as directed, faithfully. Don't quit early on because you feel better. Don't change the dosage yourself. More is not always better. Don't borrow medicine to try it out. And finally, discard old medicines (those not used within one year of purchase or whose expiration date on the label has passed). Remember, many medications can be avoided by proper lifestyle programs.

See your gynecologist at least once a year. Let him or her do a Pap smear—annually if your uterus is in, otherwise biennially. Get a mammogram faithfully each year or as indicated. Get a check for colon cancer regularly by whatever method your doctor suggests. See consultants at his or her suggestion. See your dentist and your eye doctor regularly.

Continue your HRT program. No one now knows how long or in what form your HRT will be continued. Your gynecologist will, as time goes on, undoubtedly alter and perhaps eventually discontinue it. Only time will tell.

◄§ *Pause and Reflect*

As you are now aware, aging affects our reaction to stress of all kinds—and vice versa. One of the greatest of all stresses that we face at any age is·emotional stress caused by life situations.

If we say the death of a spouse is rated as 100 on our stress scale, then what values, relative to that, do other stressful situations have?

Divorce: 70
Death of a close family member: 63
Jail: 63
Major personal injury or illness: 53

Getting fired: 47
Retirement: 45
Sexual problems: 39
Death of a close friend: 37
In-law troubles: 29

The list goes on.

Many items in this list can be avoided by proper coping mechanisms. Some, of course, cannot. Thus, the loss of a spouse is unavoidable and devastating stress. On the other hand, many illnesses and injuries can be avoided or minimized by proper planning and preventive care. Sexual problems are more readily managed today with HRT and counseling. And, in-laws at the Master life level are gone or at least governable!

The incidence of depression is increasing worldwide. No one knows why, but it is a fact. Here are some interesting things you may want to know about depression:

• A major episode of depression in a woman born in the 1930s will most likely occur as she nears fifty. However, if depression occurs in a woman born in the 1950s, it will most likely happen when she is about thirty.

• Although experts have long pooh-poohed the notion that estrogen and testosterone have any value in the management of depression, it has recently been established that such is the case. These steroid sex hormones play a distinct role in the control of related depressive problems.

• An interesting study, initiated by the National Institute of Mental Health, provided three separate categories of treatment at various institutions for depressed patients. The first two groups were exposed to two different types of psychotherapy, the third to antidepressant drug therapy or an inert placebo. The results? The drug therapy worked more rapidly and more effectively than psychotherapy. The placebo failed, but not completely. While the three groups each eventually had about a 60 percent cure rate, the placebo helped almost 30 percent of those who took it.

Outward Bound is an organization that dumps acceptable volunteer groups or individuals—for a price—into the wilderness with a minimum of equipment and a maximum of advice. The game is to get back to civilization intact and self-confident. Master Citizens, who are mainly self-confident to begin with, are accepted for this program when they qualify. Many older people participate simply to prove their independence and enjoy doing it.

A popular misconception is that earlier generations were far more devoted to their elders than children are today. This stereotype is just not true. For instance:

• About 78% of all adults over eighty-five live in their own homes or with relatives.

• An estimated 5 million Americans provide parental care in some way on any given day.

• Over 70% of the 2.2 million Americans who provide care to the frail elderly are women (23% are wives, 29% daughters, 19% other females). Their average age is fifty-seven, but fully one-third of them are over sixty-five. Of the daughters who provide care, 44% work outside of their homes, while

11% percent quit work to provide full-time care. Nearly one-third are poor—or near poor.

The enormous sacrifices that these caregivers are making has only recently been recognized. Their efforts to make living as normal as possible for aging relatives deserves our recognition and respect.

The United Nations Vienna International Plan of Action on Aging in 1982 proposed ten basic principles to be observed for the care of the elderly, namely:

Equality, individuality, independence, choice, mobility, productivity, home-care, access to services, cohesion among generations and promotion of self-care and family care.

Even the narrowest achievement of these goals will require a great deal of energy and money, which is often channeled elsewhere. For instance, developed nations spent about $345 billion on military matters in 1978 and, during the same year, about $213 billion on health goals. Developing countries, on the other hand, spent $102 billion on arms and only $22 billion on health care matters!

It is worth noting that the United States contributed .23%—less than one-quarter of one percent—of the gross national product for the development of the aging care goals to the United Nations Organization for Economic Cooperation and Development. That represents the *lowest* contribution of *any developed nation.* The highest (1.02%) was from the Netherlands, followed by Norway (.99%) and Denmark (.85%). Saudia Arabia and Kuwait, the two grand champions of OPEC, contributed 3.5% and 4.5%, respectively, of their gross national products to provide the same assistance to other developing countries in their sphere of influence.

Your chances of living to be one hundred are about 1 in 1,000 if you live in the United States. More women live to be centenarians than do men and their chances are greatest in Hawaii (1,713 in 100,000), Minnesota (1,444), South Dakota (1,392), Iowa (1,379), Nebraska (1,364), North Dakota (1,362), Kansas (1,339), Florida (1,336), Idaho (1,329) and Arizona (1,317).

Questions
and Answers

Where does the word "menopause" come from?

In 1812 the French gynecologist C.P.L. Gardanne wrote a monograph dealing in its entirety with the change of life. In it he coined the word "ménépausie," which he derived from two Greek words meaning "month" and "terminate."

When does the menopause start?

Usually the menopause starts in the mid-forties, but there are wide variations.

Can I predict when the menopause will start?

The onset of menopause can be predicted only when your ovaries must be removed for some serious disorder. The menopause will begin the next day no matter what your age. Otherwise there is no way to know when it will begin.

What sets it off?

The decline of ovarian hormone secretion.

How will I know when I have entered the menopause?

By the onset of a group of symptoms usually including hot flashes (flushes), night sweats, insomnia, depression, fatigue and other seemingly unrelated symptoms. Sooner or later there will also be changes in your menstrual function, changes that can be variable.

How will my doctor know I have entered the menopause?

By listening to your account of your symptoms and by certain blood tests.

What is the perimenopause?

It is a descriptive term for the few years immediately preceding the menopause. During this time, the premenstrual syndrome (PMS) may be accentuated and prolonged and certain metabolic changes, such as stepped-up calcium loss, may also begin.

When does the perimenopause start?

Usually 2 to 3 years before the menopause.

When does it end?

It folds into the menopause.

Is there a distinct line between the menopause and the perimenopause?

None at all. They are a continuum.

Why does premature menopause occur?

Any condition that prematurely stops the ovaries from making estrogen will induce a premature menopause. So the premature destruction of the ovaries by disease or infection or the premature surgical removal of the ovaries for whatever reason will induce an early menopause. Certain inherited disorders as well as some severe systemic illnesses will also accomplish the same thing.

How do I know if premature menopause is happening to me?

You will have the typical signs and symptoms of the menopause.

What is the difference between temporary ovarian failure and permanent ovarian failure?

Temporary failure can occur under periods of stress and illness. By definition, recovery will occur when the offending condition is corrected. Permanent ovarian failure is, as the name suggests, an irreversible cessation of ovarian function for whatever reason.

Will the menopause be as uncomfortable as I hear it will be?

That depends on what you hear and the circumstances of your own menopause. Generally speaking, though, almost all disturbing menopausal problems can be safely and effectively controlled with adequate hormone replacement.

How does PMS relate to the menopause?

Generally PMS symptoms, if present at all, become somewhat accentuated and prolonged as the menopause draws near.

How does a hysterectomy affect the menopause?

A hysterectomy (an operation that removes the uterus only) stops all menstrual flow permanently and produces permanent sterility. It has no direct effect on the menopause except that all problems related to the bleeding certainly cease.

How will the menopause affect my sex life?

Most commonly there is a gradual decline in sex drive, sex fantasy and vaginal lubrication along with an increase in time-to-orgasm. In later, postmenopausal years the vagina becomes very thin and dry, making sexual intercourse painful. All this assumes there has been no hormone replacement.

Do I need to continue using birth control during the menopause?

You need to practice birth control until you have not menstruated for one year. Special circumstances (hormone replacement, for instance) may alter that rule. Your doctor will know.

What role do oral contraceptives play in the menopause?

Under the proper conditions, birth control pills may be used at the menopause not only as a contraceptive but also as a menopausal hormone supplement. Mainly, to use birth control pills you must not smoke, should not have significant hypertension and must have a satisfactory experience with both their menopausal and birth control effects.

Will I gain weight during the menopause?

You can, but it will most likely be due to other body changes that occur in the middle years. Men have middle-age spread, too, but don't have a menopause. Almost anything that happens during the menopause is blamed on the menopause.

How often should I see my doctor during the menopause?

If there are no specific medical problems related to the menopause or some other gynecological condition, once a year is adequate. Otherwise, your doctor will advise you.

Do you recommend any annual tests?

A vaginal Pap smear should be performed and, during your fifties, an annual mammogram is necessary. Certain other tests may be required at regular intervals but under special circumstances and not necessarily on an annual basis.

How important is hormone replacement therapy?

It is less important than insulin for a diabetic, but it is probably as important as any replacement therapy that you might ever be involved with.

Isn't hormone replacement therapy filled with risks?

No, it is not. In ordinary circumstances, the benefits vastly outweigh the few risks involved.

How is hormone replacement administered?

It may be given orally as tablets, by injection under the skin either by shots or pellets, or across the skin (transdermally), using abdominal patches or vaginal creams.

How far into the menopause should I start hormone replacement therapy?

As soon as you have symptoms.

Will hormone therapy help to stabilize my mood swings?

Yes.

How much does hormone replacement therapy cost?

Depending on what method you use and whether or not you substitute generic products, from $10.00 to $20.00 per month.

Should I continue hormone replacement after the menopause?

Yes. For how long, however, depends upon many factors only you and your doctor can resolve.

Should I take vitamins during the menopause?

You are probably asking about combination vitamin and mineral preparations. Most diets adequately provide most vitamins and minerals, but you need to be sure that you have a little extra iron until menstruation ceases and that you take a calcium supplement always. An ordinary once-a-day vitamin supplement is very adequate and, after menstruation ceases, just a once-a-day vitamin pill plus a calcium supplement.

What is the postmenopause?

These are the years that follow the more or less acute time of the menopause, when menses are about to end and when the many other symptoms related to the menopause (flushing and so on) have largely abated or disappeared.

When does the postmenopause start?

As noted above, when the acute menopause phase subsides.

When does it end?

It doesn't end—rather, it continues.

Is there a distinct line between the menopause and post-menopause?

No. The one flows slowly into the other as the perimenopause flows into the menopause.

What role does estrogen play in the postmenopausal years?

In most instances it has an important role in maintaining bone strength, delaying hardening of the arteries and supporting vaginal health as well as sexual drive.

What role does progesterone play in the postmenopause?

It continues to protect the uterus and, perhaps, the breasts against the unopposed irritation that estrogen by itself has upon these organs. Further, it may help build new bone.

How are estrogen and progesterone interrelated?

They are both secreted from maturing egg follicles in the ovary and are very closely related steroid hormones.

How will a lack of estrogen affect me physically and emotionally?

Without estrogen, menses cease and the vagina atrophies. Equally, the breasts atrophy as does the skin. The rate of bone loss accelerates and the rate of arterial hardening increases. Emotionally, depression increases and sex drive decreases. Hot flushes and emotional instability along with fatigue and many other general systemic complaints become the rule.

How does testosterone figure into the hormone replacement program?

Testosterone (the male hormone) is a sexual stimulant for both men and women. Healthy ovaries secrete testosterone-like hormones, which act as a sexual stimulant. After the menopause, these hormones are often not present, and so testosterone is added to certain hormone replacement programs to supply this need.

How does nutrition affect the whole menopausal-post-menopausal complex?

Proper nutrition is always important. During these times in . a woman's life, however, an adequate diet is even more important. Your food must supply most basic needs and your supplements, the rest. Animal fats and salt must be restricted to help avoid hypertension and other vascular disease and, finally, the number of calories must be decreased as body needs decrease so that obesity does not follow.

How is exercise important in the whole menopausal-post-menopausal complex?

Proper exercise plays many roles at this time. It helps in maintaining bone strength, it burns off excess calories and it vastly improves cardio-pulmonary strength and reserves. It also promotes a sense of well-being at any time.

How can I tell if I am at risk for osteoporosis?

Factors that promote the onset of osteoporosis include a family history of the condition, a very early menopause, a thin body, a fair complexion, an inactive lifestyle, an alcohol or tobacco habit and an inadequate diet. There are a few others, but these are the main risk factors.

How can I prevent osteoporosis?

By an adequate diet, including a proper calcium intake, an active, ongoing exercise program, avoidance of tobacco and alcohol and hormone replacement as indicated.

What role does calcium play in osteoporosis?

Adequate calcium intake is necessary to keep up with calcium loss. Bones lose calcium very rapidly in the early years of the menopause and postmenopause. It must be replaced. However, calcium supplementation is useless at this time without accompanying estrogen.

What are my chances of developing a breast disorder?

You have about a 50-50 chance of developing some minor breast disorder. Fortunately, however, breast cancer—the most serious breast disorder—will occur in just about 10 percent of all women today. That is still much too high a figure, but great hope of abatement is on the horizon.

How important are mammograms?

Just about as important as breathing. At this moment, only mammograms done as and when directed by the American Cancer Society can arrest this most disabling female cancer. Regular mammograms and Pap smears are so important to you that it is hard to equate them in importance with anything else you may do.

Outtakes

Perimenopause (PeriMPX)

Definition: A period of time immediately preceeding the true menopause, when certain menopausal characteristics may appear.

Cause: The beginning decline of ovarian function.

Time frame: Usually two or three years' duration.

Symptoms: An increase in the intensity and/or duration of premenstrual syndrome (PMS), fatigue, rarely premenstrual flushing, sometimes declining sexual interest.

Progression: PeriMPX symptoms generally increase as menopause approaches.

Diagnosis: Usually by patient's symptoms. Sometimes cessation of ovulation can be determined by certain tests.

Treatment: Medical management of PMS symptoms, hormone replacement therapy (HRT) if necessary, lifestyle changes, including diet and exercise, and counseling.

Outcome: Good response to adequate therapy and advancement into the menopause.

Menopause (MPX)

Definition: The time of cessation of menstruation and the emotional and physical changes that accompany it.

Cause: The cessation of ovarian function and, thus, of hormone production.

Time frame: Usually between age forty-five and fifty-five and lasting several years.

Symptoms: Irregularity in, and finally absence of, menstrual bleeding, along with flushes, sweats, insomnia, depression, irritability, headaches, palpitations and numerous other less-common symptoms.

Diagnosis: Through patient's history, laboratory tests for declining estrogen production, absence of ovulation and elevated pituitary levels of follicle stimulating hormone (FSH).

Treatment: Hormone replacement therapy when physician and patient agree and when therapy is not contraindicated, plus counseling in diet, exercise and many other aspects of mature living.

Outcome: Gradual and peaceful progression into the postmenopausal years.

Postmenopause (PMPX)

Definition: All of the years following the acute menopausal events.

Cause: Virtually complete absence of the ovarian hormones, estrogen and progesterone.

Time frame: As indicated above—all the years following the menopause.

Symptoms and signs: Increasingly rapid arteriosclerosis (hardening of the arteries), osteoporosis with all its bony frame damage, declining sexual drive and thinning of the vaginal lining, which results in lubrication failure and, often, painful lovemaking.

Diagnosis: Through continuing high blood FSH levels along with low estrogen levels, low vaginal estrogen smears, evidence of increasing arteriosclerosis and osteoporosis, patient's symptoms.

Management: HRT, calcium supplementation, diet, exercise and adequate counseling.

Outcome: A gentle and safe journey into maturity.

Glossary

Words in SMALL CAPITAL LETTERS are also entries in this glossary.

Adrenal glands: ENDOCRINE glands that secrete hormones into the body. The adrenal hormones are mainly adrenalin and CORTISONE, but the glands are also capable of making a TESTOSTERONE-like hormone. There is an adrenal gland sitting on top of each kidney.

amenorrhea: The absence of MENSTRUATION.

androstenedione: A hormone substance made in the ADRENAL GLANDS and in the OVARIES. It resembles the male hormone TESTOSTERONE in many of its actions.

anemia: A decrease in the red blood cell count below acceptable limits. Anemia may be due to blood loss, an iron-deficient diet or a number of systemic disorders.

arteriosclerosis: The deposition of calcium plaques along the arterial walls, also known as hardening of the arteries. This aging process is accelerated by high cholesterol blood levels and by smoking.

breast self-examination: The technique of examining one's own breasts. The technique, which should be done monthly, may be learned from a physician, from mammogram clinics, hospital wellness centers and pamphlets put out by the American Cancer Society and other agencies.

calcium: A mineral element fundamental for normal body function. The daily diet should include 1000 mg of calcium in order to satisfy bone, muscle and blood needs.

calcitonin: A hormone secreted by the parafollicular cells of the THYROID GLAND, another ENDOCRINE organ. Calcitonin is important in regulating the storage of CALCIUM in bone.

climacteric: Another term for the MENOPAUSE. The term is not very popular, so it is not used very often.

corpus luteum: A mass of hormone-secreting tissue in the ovary. After OVULATION occurs, the granulosal cells that surrounded the maturing egg and made ESTROGEN are converted to lutein cells and begin to secrete PROGESTERONE. These remnant cells remain organized in a cyst-like cavity called the corpus luteum ("yellow body"). The whole structure disintegrates just before MENSTRUA- TION.

cortical bone: Thick, smooth, hard plates of dense bone, as opposed to honey-combed TRABECULAR bone. The outside long shafts of the bones in our extremities are perfect examples of cortical bone.

cortisone: A very powerful hormone secreted from the ADRENAL GLANDS and needed for the proper function of many body systems. It is often used in medicine to treat serious disorders of body function, certain auto-immune diseases, some arthritis and serious allergic disorders.

endocrine glands: Glands that secrete hormones internally. The hormones then go somewhere else to do their work. Included here are the ADRENALS, OVARIES and testicles, THYROID, PARA-THYROID, PITUITARY and certain others.

endometriosis: A disorder of the pelvic organs where little blood cysts made up of ENDOMETRIUM cells are found on the uterus, tubes, ovaries, pelvic ligaments and even bladder and bowel wall. It is a painful condition because these little blood cysts menstruate internally each month and grow a little bigger. It is associated with infertility.

endometrium: The normal lining of the uterine cavity that grows each month under the influence of ESTROGEN and PROGESTER-ONE and then partially menstruates away unless pregnancy has occurred.

estradiol (E2): One of the two main ESTROGENS. Almost all E2 is made within the ovary.

estrogen: The basic female hormone produced by the OVARIES in a monthly pattern throughout the reproductive years. An integral part of HRT (hormone replacement therapy).

estrone (E1): One of the two main ESTROGENS. It is largely made from ESTRADIOL (E2).

flushes: In the MENOPAUSE, a feeling of heat and warmth, beginning somewhere deep inside and resulting in a flushed and red face. An individual flush lasts several minutes.

follicle stimulating hormone (FSH): One of several PITUITARY hormones that stimulates the OVARIES. Each month FSH initiates maturation of a capable follicle so that it prepares for OVULATION. FSH also stimulates the granulosal cells in each maturing follicle to make ESTROGEN.

hormone replacement therapy (HRT): When the ovaries cease to function adequately, or if they have been removed surgically,

HRT with proper amounts of ESTROGEN and PROGESTERONE is given to fill the void created.

hormone smear: A test used to determine estrogen levels in the body. Estrogen stimulates the vaginal lining to grow, and it maintains the lining in a mature, healthy state. Smears taken from the vaginal wall and stained reveal the degree of maturity, and a count of these scraped-off cells is called a maturation index. This index is a general indicator of estrogen levels in the body.

hysterectomy: The removal of the uterus, whether done abdominally or vaginally.

luteinizing hormone (LH): A powerful PITUITARY hormone that surges out somewhere around the middle of a regular menstrual cycle. It forces the mature follicle to OVULATE and stimulates development of the CORPUS LUTEUM. Modern home ovulation-predictor kits can identify this LH surge and thus predict ovulation a few hours before it happens.

mammography: An x-ray technique that, using very minimal radiation, detects serious breast disease at a much earlier time and with much greater accuracy than any other single or combined examination or test.

mastectomy: The surgical removal of a breast. A radical mastectomy is the removal of a breast along with associated and surrounding muscle, gland tissues and skin.

menarche: The beginning of MENSTRUATION.

menopause (MPX): The mid-life cessation of MENSES and the attendant body changes associated with it and around it.

menses: See MENSTRUATION.

menstruation: The regular monthly flow of blood and tissue debris from the uterus.

MPX: A common abbreviation signifying MENOPAUSE.

myomata: Fibrous muscular tumors that quite commonly grow upon and within the uterine walls. Almost always benign, these tumors may get very large and may cause heavy, painful uterine bleeding. Also commonly called *fibroids.*

night sweats: Hot flashes that occur during the night. Usually the intense heat makes you push your covers back and you awaken cooled by the sweat evaporating on your now-exposed skin.

osteoporosis: A condition characterized by the decrease in bone mass that results in frailty of the bones. When CALCIUM leaves bone, for whatever reason, the bone becomes weakened and osteoporosis exists. There are many causes of osteoporosis, simple aging being one of them. The loss of ESTROGEN at the MENO-PAUSE, however, is by far the commonest and most serious cause of osteoporosis. Without estrogen, calcium leaves the bone at a very rapid rate.

ovary: The female sex gland. The ovaries are responsible for more or less regular OVULATION and for the secretion of ESTROGEN, PROGESTERONE and certain other hormones into the circulation.

ovulation: The releasing of an egg from the OVARY into the peritoneal cavity, which surrounds or encloses all abdominal organs.

oxytocin: A PITUITARY hormone that affects the reproductive organs. Oxytocin makes the uterine muscle contract vigorously. Thus it is important during labor. This hormone also helps initiate lactation.

Pap smear: A smear taken from the uterine cervix, stained and examined in a way perfected by a Greek-born American anatomist, George Papanicolaou. This smear, taken on a regular basis, has saved millions of women from cancer of the cervix. At present there is a virtual epidemic of cancer of the cervix in our youngsters. This is due to the widespread presence of the human papilloma virus (HPV) in the teenage population. It is a sexually transmitted virus that lives in the vagina and cervix and in the male's sexual anatomy. It is very important, then, that all sexually active youngsters have regular (at least annual) Pap smears.

parathyroid glands: A series of tiny ENDOCRINE GLANDS lying behind the THYROID. They secrete substances that control CALCIUM metabolism and balance.

perimenopause (PeriMPX): The two- to three-year period before the menopause, when some signs of declining hormone production begin to appear. The PREMENSTRUAL SYNDROME, for instance, should it be present, tends to intensify. These years, for descriptive and clinical purposes, have been designated the PeriMPX.

pituitary gland: The master ENDOCRINE GLAND. Its secretions control and effect all the other glands and many basic body functions. Much of this gland's power remains a mystery.

postmenopause (PMPX): After the more or less acute years of MENSES cessation and after the visceral symptoms (FLUSHES, for example) subside, the postmenopause begins. And it comprises all the years that follow.

premature menopause: The cessation of MENSES before forty accompanied by typical menopausal symptoms. There are many causes.

premature ovarian failure: As the name suggests, the failure of the ovaries to function prior to the established time of MENOPAUSE. This may be temporary and due to stress of various sorts or severe illnesses—but recovery is the rule. Or it may be permanent and become a premature menopause. There are several causes.

premenstrual syndrome (PMS): A very complex set of disorders that precedes MENSTRUATION by a variable number of days. Depression, irritability, swelling, breast tenderness, headaches and many other symptoms characterize this common condition. The treatment is varied and not uniformly successful.

primary osteoporosis: Bone loss that occurs with aging or with ESTROGEN deficiency.

progestagens: Synthetic hormones that resemble PROGESTERONE closely, both in their chemical makeup and in their effects upon the female body. Also called progestins.

progesterone: An important female hormone produced in the OVARIES. It is secreted by lutein cells found in the CORPUS LUTEUM cyst, which is a normal structure formed at the site of OVULATION and which has a lifespan of about two weeks. It is important for normal MENSTRUATION, for the maintenance of pregnancy (if one should occur, the corpus luteum lives on) and to combat the irritative action of ESTROGEN on the ENDOMETRIUM and other tissues.

progestin: See PROGESTAGENS.

prolactin: A hormone made by the PITUITARY gland. Normally, it supports lactation, but when overproduced by certain pituitary abnormalities, it can arrest all menstrual function.

secondary osteoporosis: The form of bone weakening and demineralization that is always secondary to some other disorder. Many glandular and bone diseases can produce this form of bone weakness.

steroids: Variations of a chemical configuration made by the body from cholesterol that result in all the sex hormones and most adrenal hormones.

temporary ovarian failure: The shutting down or diminishing of ovarian function for a period of time. Stress—such as that caused by excessive exercise, bulemia or anorexia and life situations of many kinds—can halt ovarian activity for a period of time. Moreover, many severe illnesses can do the same thing. As the term implies, ovarian recovery will follow removal of the cause.

testosterone: The male hormone secreted by the testicles and, perhaps, in small amounts, by certain other tissues in both men and women.

thenarche: The beginning of breast buds and breast development. This usually precedes the menarche (beginning of MEN-STRUATION) by a few years.

thyroid gland: As part of the ENDOCRINE system, the thyroid gland secretes thyroid hormone into the bloodstream, and this hormone regulates all body metabolism. The thyroid gland also secretes CALCITONIN, which helps control CALCIUM activity in the body.

trabecular bone: The honey-combed bone girders found inside the firm shafts of exterior CORTICAL BONE. Look in the center of the bone in a T-bone steak and you will see trabecular bone.

Index

About the Author

Dr. Gillespie was born in North Bay, Ontario, Canada, and educated at McGill University in Montreal. His training in obstetrics and gynecology was completed in the United States and he now lives and practices in Little Rock, Arkansas. Dr. Gillespie is certified by the American Board of Obstetrics and Gynecology and is a Fellow of the American College of Obstetricians and Gynecologists. In 1977 he was elected a Fellow of the Royal College of Obstetricians and Gynecologists in London, England, an unusual honor for American citizens. Besides maintaining his private practice he serves as clinical professor of obstetrics and gynecology at the University of Arkansas School of Medicine. He is a member of a number of scientific societies and has received awards for his research from the American Medical Association, the Southern Medical Association, the American Fertility Society and the Pacific Coast Fertility Society.

Dr. Gillespie is the author of numerous scientific publications, as well as *Your Pregnancy Month by Month* and *Prime-life Pregnancy*.